Militarized Maternity

Militarized Maternity

EXPERIENCING PREGNANCY
IN THE U.S. ARMED FORCES

Megan D. McFarlane

UNIVERSITY OF CALIFORNIA PRESS

University of California Press
Oakland, California

© 2021 by Megan D. McFarlane

Library of Congress Cataloging-in-Publication Data

Names: McFarlane, Megan, author.
Title: Militarized maternity : experiencing pregnancy in the U.S. armed forces / Megan D. McFarlane.
Description: Oakland, California : University of California Press, [2021] | Includes bibliographical references and index.
Identifiers: LCCN 2020043906 (print) | LCCN 2020043907 (ebook) | ISBN 9780520344686 (cloth) | ISBN 9780520344693 (paperback) | ISBN 9780520975620 (epub)
Subjects: LCSH: Women soldiers—United States. | Pregnancy—United States. | Maternal and infant welfare—United States.
Classification: LCC UB418.W65 M375 2021 (print) |
 LCC UB418.W65 (ebook) | DDC 355.1/20820973—dc23
LC record available at https://lccn.loc.gov/2020043906
LC ebook record available at https://lccn.loc.gov/2020043907

30 29 28 27 26 25 24 23 22 21
10 9 8 7 6 5 4 3 2 1

To Steven, Evelyn, and Theodore

Contents

	Acknowledgments	ix
1.	Examining the Pregnancy Continuum in the U.S. Military	1
2.	Contextualizing Military Maternity Experiences	23
3.	Hyperplanning Pregnancies	40
4.	Performing Macho Maternity	71
5.	Negotiating Postpartum Policies	99
6.	Redefining Military Maternity	146
	Appendix A Research Participants: Demographics	165
	Appendix B Profiles: Enlisted Servicewomen	167
	Appendix C Profiles: Female Officers	171
	Notes	179
	Bibliography	217
	Index	239

Acknowledgments

It's often said that it takes a village to raise a child. I, and the many women interviewed for this book, agree this is true. I would also argue it also takes a village to write a book. Thanks to my village, this book has changed and evolved in all the best ways. The earliest version started as a chapter in my dissertation. Iterations of chapters 1, 2, and 3 were published in *Women's Studies in Communication*, and later drafts of those chapters were presented at annual conventions of the National Communication Association. In what follows, I do my best to thank my village for influencing many of the changes that led to this eventual book project.

First and foremost, thank you to all of the amazing servicewomen who were willing to share your inspiring stories with me, many of which are included in this book. I am indebted to you. (All of the names of interviewed servicewomen are pseudonyms.)

Thank you to the Organization for Women and Communication (ORWAC) and Marymount University for their generous grants that helped fund this project in important ways.

Thank you to Lyn Uhl, executive editor at University of California Press, who saw this project as important and whose guidance and encouragement made the process much easier. Thank you to Naomi Schneider, UCP executive editor, who has helped guide this project to its finish. Thank you also to the two reviewers who asked thoughtful questions, pushed me, and were willing to read and give feedback during a pandemic.

Thank you to my mentors. Thank you to Heather Canary, Kevin DeLuca, Ella Myers, Kent Ono, Sarah Projansky, and Helene Shugart for all of your thoughts and insights at the earliest stages of this project. To Tom Carmody, who introduced me to rhetorical criticism and has continued to encourage me in the years since then. To Robin Jensen, for teaching me how to write with coherence, for talking with me about reproductive justice, and for exchanging many stories about our children and being working mothers. To Marouf Hasian Jr., for teaching me the importance of abundant citations, bringing me on to your projects, making me find my own answers and my own plan, and always supporting me in my decisions. And to Cindy Griffin, who has been supporting and encouraging me since I sought your feedback as an undergraduate student who was citing your work, and without whom this book project would likely have taken a much longer time to see the light of day. Our chats have been invaluable bright spots for me, as well.

Thank you to my academic friends who have become my lifelong friends: Betsy Brunner, Veronica Dawson, and Mindy Krakow; you have been great convention roommates, running partners, editors, substitute instructors, support systems, and sounding boards.

Thank you to my family. To my parents for telling me for as long as I can remember that I can be anything, and to my mom for showing me what it is to be a working mother who can have a successful career while raising kids.

Thank you to Steven, Evelyn, and Theodore. Evy was five months old when I started interviewing servicewomen, and Theo was born shortly before I started my second round of interviews with female officers. Their births, and my experience as a working mom after they were born, inspired, informed, and influenced this project in significant and important ways. Throughout the entire process, which predates this book project, Steve has provided continuous love, support, encouragement, and a listening ear. I am incredibly grateful we get to go through life together.

1 Examining the Pregnancy Continuum in the U.S. Military

> People were like "Oh, isn't it hard being a woman in the military?" and I'm like "You know, I bet it's harder for a woman at a bank or at a law firm, where she has to negotiate these same gender issues, but she has no one fighting for her."
>
> —Elizabeth*

In the summer of 2012, several events related to women's maternity experiences sparked public conversations in the United States about (in)appropriate maternal behavior. Kicking it off was an image of Jamie Lynne Grumet, a slender twenty-six-year-old mother in skinny jeans, featured on the cover of *Time* magazine's May 21, 2012, issue breastfeeding her three-year-old son with the headline, "Are You Mom Enough?" Grumet, standing with one hand on her hip, and the other around her son, looks directly at the camera, defiantly. Her son is standing on a chair to reach his mother's breasts, wearing camouflage pants, hands hanging by his sides. He is simultaneously attempting to look at the camera while nursing from his mother's breast. Many found the picture of Grumet and her son to be extreme and shocking.[1]

A few months later, in August of 2012, a second picture circulated that featured two U.S. Air Force women in combat uniform

---

* Elizabeth is a pseudonym. All the servicewomen interviewed for this project either chose or were given pseudonyms to protect their privacy. Profiles of the interviewees are included in appendixes B and C.

1

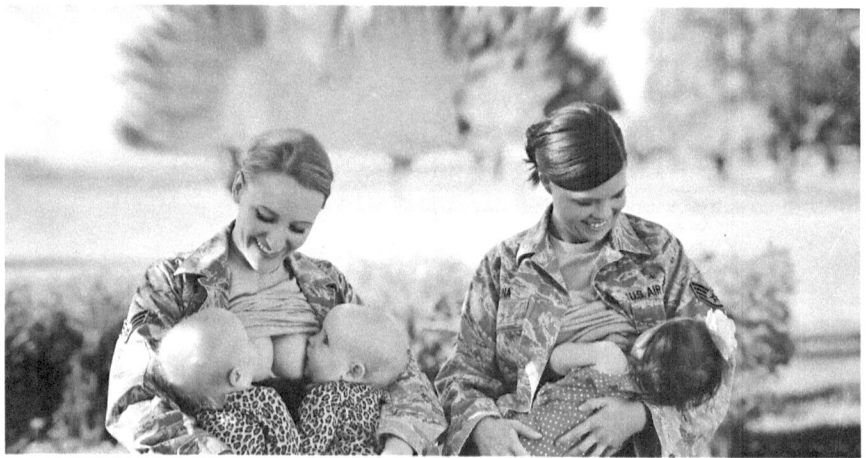

Figure 1.1. Image circulated by Mom2Mom support group to promote World Breastfeeding Week 2012. Image used with permission of Brynja Sijurdardottir.

breastfeeding their babies (figure 1.1). First shared on social media by the Mom2Mom support group in order to promote World Breastfeeding Week, the picture shows two U.S. Air Force servicewomen sitting in a field or park. Both women have their hair pulled back into tight buns, are wearing makeup, and their uniform jackets are unbuttoned to accommodate nursing their children. Terran Echegoyen-McCabe is featured on the left, breastfeeding her ten-month-old twin girls, while Christina Luna is on the right nursing her toddler. Whereas Luna's daughter is positioned in front of her left breast, concealing her body, Echegoyen-McCabe's breasts are quite visible, as her shirt has to be pulled up much farther to accommodate feeding two babies simultaneously. The result is an image of Echegoyen-McCabe's generous cleavage, since her body is unconcealed. The picture of Echegoyen-McCabe and Luna generated significant controversy, with some arguing the image was as offensive as urinating or defecating on the military uniform.[2]

Between these photographic events, Marissa Mayer became CEO of Yahoo in July 2012, when she was pregnant and expecting a son in September. Shortly after accepting the position, Mayer announced that she would take only one or two weeks of maternity leave after the birth of her son and that, while she was gone, she would continue to work from home.[3] Soon after returning from her fleeting maternity leave, Mayer announced that Yahoo would no longer allow telecommuting, a flexible work arrangement many new mothers—and new parents in general—appreciate.

Following these events, in early 2013, Sheryl Sandberg, the chief operating officer of Facebook, released her book, *Lean In*. In it, she encouraged women in the workforce, and especially male-dominated organizations, to "lean in" to opportunities and be more assertive. She also argued that women should not "leave before you leave"—meaning that sometimes, when working women want to have babies, they start to close doors of opportunities, believing that they cannot be successful at work and at home.[4]

Each of these instances generated public discussions and debates about what constitutes (in)appropriate behavior for pregnant women and mothers. And, with the exception of the *Time* magazine cover, they also brought the concept of what it means to be good *working* mothers front and center.[5] Because of the patriarchal foundations of organizations in general, and male-dominated organizations especially, female workers in tech firms (like Yahoo and Facebook) and the military have historically faced professional challenges related to gender and power, making the focus on women's maternity even more complex.[6] Whereas discussions of Mayer and Sandberg focused on the work-life balance of the two working mothers, conversations around the picture of the two servicewomen breastfeeding in uniform focused primarily on whether or not it was appropriate to publicly breastfeed in a military uniform.[7] I argue, however, that the image is about being a working mother in the U.S. military and that the controversy stirred up by the image of two women breastfeeding in military uniforms revealed how little is known or understood about the maternity experiences of active-duty servicewomen in the U.S. armed forces.

It was when I saw the image of Echegoyen-McCabe and Luna breastfeeding in uniform and read the comments in response to it that this research project initially began. I was curious about the strong negative responses, and wanted to understand why people found it so extremely offensive.[8] This research then led me to ask more questions about servicewomen's maternity experiences in general, specifically (a) What kind of culture do the discursive practices around pregnancy and maternity in the U.S. military construct? And, (b) in what ways do servicewomen comply with and/or resist this construction and with what consequences? Ultimately, what I discovered is that, although the military is explicitly working to accommodate the reality of motherhood (by offering extensive maternity leave, space and time for pumping, and other policies that will be further discussed in this book), the overall culture of the military in which maternity is seen as a problem has not changed. This policy/culture disconnect is so ingrained that even pregnant servicewomen have internalized it and often perpetuate the discriminatory culture themselves. Therefore, I argue that unless the problematic culture surrounding maternity in the military is challenged, these policy changes will not be as effective as they should be at reducing pregnancy discrimination in the military.

To reach these conclusions, I had to adjust my research methods. Up to that point in my academic career, I had been trained in rhetorical analysis; yet it quickly became apparent that conducting a rhetorical analysis of traditional discourses, such as policies, newspaper stories, and military documents, would not be enough; I was still missing a large piece of the puzzle: the voices of the stakeholders. To be sure, I would have learned much about pregnancy culture in the U.S. military by looking at those documents, but the voices of those most affected would still not be heard, and I would be contributing to their misrepresentation and to the pattern of devaluing their voices. Ultimately, efforts to answer my research questions would require expanding my methods.

PIECING THE PUZZLE TOGETHER:
NOTES ON METHOD

In order to create a more nuanced cultural context in which to understand servicewomen's maternity experiences, I employ a critical feminist orientation that draws from others who have combined interviews with extant rhetorical analysis.[9] This approach asserts that rhetoric is not a singular product to be analyzed, such as a speech, but rather is a collection of texts and discourses that create a larger context.[10] In this view, discourse to be examined may include linguistic symbols (e.g., policies, documents, speeches, words) and material symbols (e.g., bodies, photographs, art)—the discursive fragments or puzzle pieces that contribute to the larger puzzle/context under analysis.[11] By referring to these discursive fragments as "rhetorical," I echo Britt, in order to emphasize that these puzzle pieces "present a point of view, help constitute identities, and influence thought and action."[12] To be sure, rhetoric is consequential. It is not passive or neutral; it is a constructive power that is always politically and ideologically invested.[13] Therefore, the goal of rhetorical analysis is to investigate, explain, and evaluate texts/puzzle pieces in order to gain a better understanding of the rhetorical processes at work, and how they are (re)constructing particular ideologies.[14]

In the case of this project, the rhetorical fragments/puzzle pieces analyzed include newspaper and magazine articles; military policies, pamphlets, brochures, and procedures; and peer-reviewed journals (both military and nonmilitary). I also conducted interviews with servicewomen who experienced pregnancy while serving on active duty in the U.S. military. I included servicewomen who were pregnant at the time, had been pregnant recently, or had experienced a pregnancy since 2001. The heightened military presence after the terrorist attacks on September 11, 2001, resulted in more military recruits and a higher number of women serving in the military.[15] Many policy changes regarding women followed suit in efforts to recruit and retain women. Some of these changes include extended maternity leave, required breastfeeding facilities, longer breaks from deployment after giving birth, increased access to abortion, and opening combat positions to women.[16] Therefore, interviewing women who served after changes were enacted provides insight about how women who have more recently served in the U.S. military have experienced pregnancy.

The inclusion of interviews follows other rhetorical scholars who use qualitative methods.[17] It is also driven by the critical feminist call to embrace what Haraway referred to as "situated knowledges," which welcome the subjective nature of lived experience to better understand how knowledge is socially constructed through discourse.[18] This type of analysis privileges women's voices to address the multiple issues and experiences and to determine how they are similar, different, or overlapping.[19] Indeed, this was the case for this research, as well. The interviews took place in two phases, using initial recruiting and snowball sampling.[20] In the first phase, I interviewed enlisted servicewomen from the Navy, Air Force, and Army. In the second phase, I interviewed current and recently retired officers in the Navy and Air Force. Because of the different qualifications for enlisted servicemembers and officers, and the related differences in jobs and responsibilities, experiences often differ greatly between enlisted servicewomen and female officers, and interviewing both gave better insight into military maternity experiences across the board. Although the nature of snowball sampling resulted in the recruitment of a majority of Navy servicewomen, participants were still fairly diverse in terms of age, branch, race, and location for the enlisted participants, and all interviews highlighted the diversity and similarity of military pregnancy experiences.[21]

Using interviews to study organizations—and maternity experiences within organizations in particular—is common in the field of communication studies.[22] Yet Cheney and Lair and others have argued for the importance of using rhetorical methods to study organizations (in this case, the military), as the discoveries can supplement findings from other research perspectives.[23] This creates what Pezzullo calls "critical interruptions," which allow for a new way of thinking and understanding, and can lead to different solutions.[24]

For example, the U.S. military has some exemplary maternity policies; yet, as the following chapters will demonstrate, despite exponential changes in maternity-related policies—from maternity leave to breastfeeding—servicewomen are still struggling to balance their families and their military careers. Often they must choose to leave the military as a way to find a manageable balance. Using rhetorical analysis as well as interviews in this case may lead to the critical interruptions not discovered by one method alone. For instance, it was through interviewing servicewomen that I had perhaps one of the largest insights/critical interruptions that influenced the organization of my research and this book. It occurred during my interview with Michelle, a retired Navy officer. I asked her specifically about her pregnancy experience as an active-duty servicemember, and she responded by noting that pregnancy experiences are not isolated to the nine months of pregnancy. Instead, as she explained, "pregnancy is sort of all rolled up together with the fact that you then have a baby and then you're a parent. So, it's hard to pull out my experiences of pregnancy with my experiences of parenting because they're all in a continuum. . . . I'm going to consider it part of the same issue." These few sentences changed how I would frame this project. My initial plan was to only discuss the actual months women were pregnant, which would only provide an extremely limited viewpoint that did not capture the larger maternity and motherhood experience related to pregnancy.[25]

MILITARY CULTURE: PROMOTING SOCIAL CHANGE

The U.S. military has a long history as a leader in social change, "a forerunner in dealing with racial and gender discrimination issues."[26] For instance, when the U.S. military was integrated in 1948, it became a model for integration in larger U.S. society. Additionally, the military is also known for employing a gender- and race-neutral pay scale. This means, as Elizabeth, a retired Navy officer, explained, that women "get equal pay for equal work." For example, if there is a male and female lieutenant serving at the same command, they earn the same salary. Michelle, a retired Navy officer, explicated,

> They say in general women are paid less than the men. In the military, we're paid exactly the same, and I really liked that, and I liked that I wore my rank and I wore my ribbons and you know where I've been and you know what I've done and you know what my position is in this organization, you don't have to look at me and go, "Are you the doctor or are you the nurse? Are you the lawyer or are you legal aid?" And maybe you'll guess wrong because of my skin color or my sex, [but] in the military, it's clear, I'm the doctor. I mean it's obvious. And I'm getting [paid] exactly what every other person of my rank and job is getting.

It is quotes like these, and the one by Elizabeth at the opening of this chapter, that many point to when supporting arguments that gender equality exists in the military.

Furthermore, since 2000, as part of what the Air Force calls "diversity and inclusion initiatives," significant military policy changes regarding breastfeeding, maternity leave, abortion, and combat have been instituted in order to foster a more appealing work environment for women.[27] Mae, an officer in the Navy, contended that "the military set the bar very high for how they treat pregnant women." Because the military has recently struggled to maintain troop numbers, creating policies that can recruit and retain women has been crucial.[28] Similarly, the U.S. civilian workforce is struggling to retain women, so these policies may serve as a model once again.[29]

Despite all this praise and the progressive policy changes, which also include a 1974 policy that ended involuntary separations from the military due to pregnancy, there is a long history of the U.S. military framing servicewomen's fertility as both negative and a "women's issue."[30] For example, a 1979 *Time* article referred to how the military was "coping" with the "pregnancy problem,"[31] and researchers Lundquist and Smith reported that "in 1982, pregnancy was such a problem for the military that the Reagan administration called a halt to recruiting women."[32] Due to the large number of women leaving the military because of changes in their families, the military was compelled to adjust policies and procedures to maintain retention. Yet, in 2009, a U.S. commander in Iraq threatened to court-martial soldiers for pregnancy in order to highlight "the importance of appropriate reproductive planning for female soldiers."[33] Although the commander claimed he was prepared to punish both women and men, the emphasis on female soldiers implies the responsibility ultimately rests with women.[34]

Indeed, the importance of *women's* fertility planning in the military is often stressed.[35] According to an article in *Military Medicine*, women's abilities to plan their pregnancies is not only of concern for the armed forces "in terms of troop readiness, deployment, and health care costs, as pregnancy during overseas deployment is a financial and operational burden for the military," but it also is a "matter of public health as unintended pregnancy can negatively impact women's and children's well-being."[36] These concerns reinforce many cultural discourses about "super moms," "intensive mothering," and "good working mothers" and confirms the degree to which social, political, and economic responsibility is placed upon the pregnant servicewomen, omitting any responsibility with regard to men.[37] As Natalie, one of the interviewed enlisted servicewomen in this study, contended, it is not as if "you just choose to get pregnant and there's no one else involved. . . . We didn't force them [men] to do that [have sex]."

Furthermore, pregnancy has historically been perceived as a threat to two of "the three Rs" of the U.S. military: readiness and retention.[38] Although policies have changed over the years to increase retention rates of pregnant servicewomen, such as eliminating involuntary discharges for pregnancy and parenthood, concerns about pregnancy's negative impact on troop readiness persist. Researchers Duke and Ames concluded, "From a military context, the specter of female soldiers and sailors becoming pregnant compromises the bodily discipline needed to maintain readiness."[39] This statement points to the military's investments in particular understandings of bodies, sexuality, and difference. A focus on sexuality "dissolves the veneer of . . . gender neutrality," a so-called goal of the military uniform.[40] Additionally, it reinforces what Buzzanell and Ellingson have referred to as the "master narrative" of maternity in the workplace, which associates pregnancy with "deviance, sexuality, the feminine, unreliability, illness, and disability."[41] Servicewomen's body differences may threaten the key principle of readiness, therefore framing pregnant servicewomen as deviant and pregnancy as problematic.

The belief that pregnancy is a significant factor impacting troop readiness lacks strong evidence. Biggs et al. persuasively argued that no research has found that pregnancy has "a direct negative impact . . . on military readiness."[42] Despite the view of many servicemembers who believe mothers are "organizational impediments," multiple sources have acknowledged that women's absenteeism is not much greater than men's.[43] For example, Thomas and Thomas found that "the amount of lost time from the job does not generally differ for men and women, even when pregnancy and postpartum convalescence leave are included as sources of lost time."[44] Because men are injured at higher rates than women, they are also periodically unavailable for service. A more likely reason for why women's bodies are problematic may be found in the U.S. military's culture of hypermasculinity and the tensions caused therein.

AT THE INTERSECTION: CAUGHT BETWEEN CONTRADICTORY CULTURES

In examining the maternity experiences of servicewomen, it became apparent to me that women in the military, and even more so mothers, occupy a liminal space, wherein they are located at the intersection of multiple competing cultures and cultural expectations.

First, pregnant servicewomen are at the intersection of hypermasculinity and female embodiment. One of the major cultural beliefs in the military is what many have called "military masculinity" or "hypermasculinity," which often relies on biology and bodies to define difference and power.[45] In its simplest form, masculinity "is the traits, behaviors, images, values, and interests associated with being a man within a given culture. It is not a natural consequence of male biology, but a set of socially constructed practices."[46] Masculinity is often defined in the negative, by what it is *not*. For example, Kimmel explained that dominant definitions of masculinity in mainstream America depend on the exclusion of others such as women, non-White men, and homosexual men.[47] Exclusion, difference (social and biological), and contrast have been the primary ways to make meaning in the Western philosophical tradition and the male-female binary has been used to "encode a hierarchal relationship or indicate a distribution of power."[48] Masculinity and masculine roles depend on femininity and roles defined as feminine for their meaning.[49] This binary relationship is even more extreme in the military, which has historically and traditionally been linked to masculinity.[50] Pateman elaborated, "Of all the male clubs and associations, it is in the military and on the battlefield that fraternity finds its most complete expression."[51] Yet the inclusion of women in the armed forces in increasing numbers and roles makes the link between masculinity and the military more complex and complicated.[52]

Part of the complication is due to the belief that increased numbers of women correlate with progress in gender equality. Enloe explained that even with the high ratios of women serving in militaries around the world—such as in Israel, Libya, Japan, and Sweden—these high percentages must be treated "with caution. They might not be evidence of contemporary 'postsexist' enlightenment."[53] Quantity does not always mean quality, and equality is much more complex. This is problematic because increasing the number of women serving in the military seems to be a sign of feminist progress, yet their acceptance therein may nonetheless perpetuate and affirm dominant masculinity. Unless militarized masculinity is challenged culturally, gender equality and a decrease in discrimination that military policies try to enact will remain elusive.

The intense existence and persistence of military masculinity and its deep historical roots place servicewomen at an intersection—in the middle of a culture of hypermasculinity (that is more than simply their place of employment, as military service seeps into many other areas of servicemembers' lives) and their embodied female existence, which places them on the opposing side of the simplistic biological binary that undergirds military hypermasculinity. Many of the difficulties that arise from this intersectional tension, as will be noted throughout this book, are that if women adopt the military masculinity mindset, they may be promoted and successful in the organization, but they are not helping change the culture. Conversely, if women choose not to adopt this type of behavior, they may not experience professional advancement.[54]

The second tension I have noted is that between community and individualism. On the one hand, the U.S. military attempts to make everyone appear uniform, lacking individual uniqueness. Servicemembers are fighting for a cause bigger than themselves. We often hear talk about the military "brotherhood" and community, and of servicemembers sacrificing their lives for each other. Yet, at the same time, the military exists within a culture of neoliberalism, a political ethos that has become increasingly prominent in the United States, and even more so in the military, which places extreme emphasis on individual responsibility.[55] Within neoliberal ideology, the concept of "responsibilization" refers to the expectation that individuals will make "prudent responsible choices to ensure a responsible, self-sufficient future."[56] Responsibilization focuses on the individual rather than the system, and it neglects "the social and political culture in which individual responsibility is embedded and experienced"; it "ignores how choices are exercised within a context of constrained freedom."[57] This culture is intensely focused on individual choices—the choice to join the military, the choice to leave the military, the choice to conceive, the choice not to become pregnant—without recognizing the ways that some of these so-called choices might actually be constrained.

Furthermore, neoliberalist discourses are often cloaked in second-wave feminist rhetoric, but the concept of choice is in actuality post-feminist discourse that places all responsibilities for social inequalities on women.[58] One significant consequence of responsibilization in a hypermasculine culture is a neoliberal form of victim-blaming.[59] The negative consequences of any individual act are attributed to the individuals who fail to make the so-called "right" or "good" choice. Bound up in the notion of responsibilization is the presumption that the individual exercises free choice and complete control over her actions, no matter how constrained those "choices" may be. Hence, servicewomen themselves are held responsible for discrimination that they face when they are pregnant. Communication scholars Hayden and O'Brien Hallstein showed how responsibilization logics apply to discourses about reproductive decision-making and women's career paths. They explain that although we live "in an era of choice," the term "choice" is actually more "complex and challenging" than it implies. Theoretically a woman may appear to have the ability to pick whichever option she wants through "rational deliberation," but in reality, her choices are shaped by multiple factors, including, but not limited to, her relationships, race, workplace policies, access to health care, developments in reproductive technology, and social norms.[60]

Third, servicewomen are located in the liminal space between the U.S. military's post-9/11 material needs—more bodies to serve in the military as recruiting goals continue to be missed—and the post-9/11 ideological needs that Fixmer-Oraiz calls, "homeland maternity."[61] In recent years, the military branches have struggled to meet their recruitment goals, to the point where it has been called a "recruitment crisis."[62] The recruitment of more women has been part of the response to this need, during a time Fixmer-Oraiz dubs "the logic of preemption."[63] She argues that the attacks on 9/11 "provided a catalyst for reanimating familiar notions of security, nation, and citizenship."[64] Out of this emerged "homeland maternity," or the concept of a deeply intertwined connection between motherhood and nation that uses the disciplining of women's bodies as a way to bring about and promote national security. In times that appear to pose significant risks to national security, and national identity, Fixmer-Oraiz argues that the logic of preemption fuels a dramatic increase in surveillance and policing, often with the focus on women's (reproductive) bodies.

This emphasis on self-surveillance and self-discipline reflects Foucault's discussion of discipline and punishment: bodies are assumed to be docile and therefore may be "subjected" and "transformed" in ways that best serve the country.[65] However, when it comes to servicewomen and maternity, the material needs of the military and the ideological needs of the nation are put in tension with one another. On the one hand, servicewomen are expected to discipline their bodies to prevent pregnancy (and therefore conform to the bodily comportment of a "good servicemember"), similar to how servicemembers can discipline their bodies to go without food and water and withstand torture. If they cannot do this, they are punished. Hence, these "disciplinary rhetorics" constitute and shape bodies through discourse.[66] On the other hand, Fixmer-Oraiz argues that in a culture of homeland maternity, women are disciplined to adopt a "neofifties gender melodrama that reinvigorated masculinist heroism and its feminine counterpart, domesticity and dependence."[67] In this paradigm, traditional gender roles are exalted, where patriotism is equated to masculine men and dependent women whose only aspirations are domestic. It is easy to see how the material need for more bodies in the military and the rise in homeland maternity ideology are simultaneously attempting to discipline servicewomen in contradictory ways, with one asking more women to join the military and work in traditionally masculine roles and fields and the other asking women to embody traditional gender roles.

In addition to being disciplined into the military culture and the culture of homeland maternity, Mack has pointed out the disciplinary nature of what she calls "maternity culture"—"contemporary discourses surrounding the maternal body."[68] She explains how these discourses function simultaneously as *rhetorics of reproduction* and *reproducing rhetorics* because they discipline women's maternal reproducing bodies and they perpetuate problematic discursive understandings—and therefore particular views of reality—in regard to maternity.[69] Often maternity culture glorifies pain and sacrifice for the benefit of children.[70] As the maternal body is continually disciplined, it reflects and sustains the logics of neoliberalism.[71] In Mack's description of maternity culture we can see overlaps with the notions of homeland maternity and the neoliberalism found in the U.S. military culture. Ultimately, these three cultural tensions—masculinity/female embodiment, community/individual, and military/homeland maternity ideologies—are intertwined, with masculinity and neoliberalism threaded throughout all of them.

TOWARD CULTURAL CHANGE

The chapters that follow illustrate how these policing powers serve a "complex social function" that essentially works to discipline servicewomen's bodies to be more like a "normal" (male) servicemember while simultaneously disciplining them to conform to maternity culture expectations.[72] This means pregnant and nursing servicewomen are pulled in contradictory directions as they are disciplined to be "normal" servicemembers and also good pregnant women and mothers.

As many critical feminist scholars have noted, "norm" is often equated with "man," which essentially pathologizes women's bodily differences, especially during pregnancy.[73] In the U.S. military context, responsibilization discourses are propagated through various channels—institutional policies, pamphlets, and news articles, as well as cultural messages from colleagues, commanders, and health care providers—and often construct pregnant servicewomen as *choosing* to deviate from the norm of the ideal servicemember, whether or not the pregnancy was actually planned. This results in victim blaming and pathologizing women's bodies. The postfeminist, neoliberal emphasis on choice, although appearing to be empowering, ultimately undermines women's very abilities to be "agentive and self-determinant."[74]

What becomes evident through the following chapters is that institutional and cultural discourses frame pregnancy and breastfeeding as problematic, despite policies that say otherwise. In fact, despite the military's exemplary maternity policies—and, indeed, explicitly supportive language about these policies—Biggs and colleagues state that pregnancy has been, and continues to be, considered one of "the most controversial of all women-related issues debated and researched in the military, with respect to morale, discipline, attrition, and readiness."[75] I argue that the reason pregnancy remains controversial is because cultural change is not accompanying or resulting from policy changes. For example, two decades ago, Guenter-Schlesinger questioned how sexual harassment could still be such a widespread problem in the military, which "has been a forerunner in dealing with racial and gender discrimination issues" and has put substantial resources toward these issues of discrimination.[76] As we know, the military has continued to work on these issues, yet the problem still persists. Following Enloe and other scholars, I argue that polices are not resulting in significant changes because of the disconnect between policies and culture.[77] In their edited volume on women in the U.S. military, Katzenstein and Reppy and others argue that a paradox exists within the institutional culture of the U.S. military.[78] The authors specifically examine sexual assault in the armed forces, and find that changing the rules does not lead to the desired outcomes because the military culture continues to condone problematic practices, in direct contradiction to policies.

To echo Johnson et al., the *existence* of policies that support women's maternity experiences should be weighed against the *effectiveness* of the policies, and the reasons for a lack of effectiveness should be evaluated.[79] Often we have difficulty evaluating such policies because we do not know how to see outside the current preemptive and prescriptive paradigm that focuses predominantly on individual responsibility. Addressing culture can be difficult, because it means addressing a systemic, not an individual, problem. As researchers Johnson et al. noted in their study of sexual harassment in higher education sciences, engineering, and medicine, when addressing cultures, it is first, "crucial to recognize that organizational cultures are not neutral; rather, they reflect the norms and values of those who are in and have been in leadership roles in the organizations, and these norms influence the formal and informal structures, organizational strategy, human resource systems, and organizational climates."[80] In the case of the U.S. military, this means a hypermasculine neoliberal culture.

Furthermore, servicewomen themselves engage in micro-practices that contribute to and perpetuate such discourses. By practicing and reinforcing responsibilization, servicewomen become cocreators in what I call the circuit of discipline in which responsibilization is institutionalized, communicated, and performed by systems and individuals in the military.[81] This creates a loop wherein women's performances enact a culture of responsibilization—even as they recognize it should be resisted—therefore affirming a problematic ideology and further marginalizing and othering pregnant and nursing servicewomen. This circuit illuminates how and why there is a difference between policy and reality. Because the U.S. military plays an influential role in directing policy involving historically disenfranchised and marginalized populations, circuits of discipline within this organization may also point to larger structural practices that shape professional women's experiences in the civilian sector when they become pregnant.

This book serves to add to our understanding of servicewomen's experiences, and specifically the embodied experiences of pregnancy and motherhood, extending previous research on women and the military.[82] In it I examine the continuum of maternity experiences—planning pregnancies, being pregnant, breastfeeding, and postpartum mothering in the U.S. military. The book also focuses on all pregnancy experiences—unplanned and planned. This is significant, because research on U.S. servicewomen has centered on unplanned pregnancies, with specific attention paid to how these pregnancies affect troop readiness.[83] This research is likely in response to statistics like those from a 2008 survey that found that 10 percent of active-duty women had an *unintended* pregnancy within the past year.[84] These rates of unintended pregnancies are 50 percent higher than rates of unplanned pregnancies in the general public.[85] Many of these studies also serve to debunk the widespread cultural belief in the military that servicewomen *choose* to become pregnant to avoid deployment. Contained within this assumption is the belief that servicewomen can control their fertility and have complete choice over when they do and do not become pregnant, yet research finds that despite this prevailing belief, a high percentage of women have unplanned pregnancies. Many of these research studies are conducted by military doctors and health care providers advocating for better reproductive health care for servicewomen.

This book also contributes to our understanding of U.S. women's maternity experiences in general when it comes to working mothers. The way communication constructs servicewomen's pregnancy and mothering subjectivities becomes even more important, given the fact that military policies have historically influenced public policies and vice versa.[86] Therefore, policies within the military should be of interest to the general public, since they may eventually impact the larger society as well. As public discussions about maternity and working mothers proliferate in public dialogues, including pictures of servicewomen breastfeeding in uniform and top female executives like Marissa Mayer and Sheryl Sandberg discussing maternity leave and work-life balance, it is imperative that we examine why pregnant and breastfeeding women working in an organization with exemplary maternity policies—in this case, the U.S. military—still face discrimination and stigmas. Policy change does not always equal culture change, because policies, are only "as effective as the culture that supports them."[87] And this becomes even more difficult if servicewomen themselves are enacting problematic cultural norms.

ENVISIONING A DIFFERENT CULTURE

I want to be clear that, although I criticize the military, the goal of this book is not to denounce it. I am aware that my feminist and critical rhetorical approach may seem incongruous with this stance. Indeed, there are clear tensions at play in my analysis, as I recognize—along with many other feminist and critical rhetorical scholars—the problems with the masculinized, hierarchical organization of the military that is always already hostile to women and to different bodies more broadly. These are problems that are inherent in the militarism and militarization of society. Yet, like many of the servicewomen I interviewed, I refuse to view the U.S. military as *either* good *or* bad, because, in addition to its problems, there are many positive aspects to the military, many ways it has positively influenced society and continues to do so, as I discuss throughout this book. An either/or approach would assert that I *either* support a critical feminist approach *or* I support the military. I disagree. I have written this book in support of *servicewomen* and a desire to understand the policy-culture disconnect in order to envision a better future. Therefore, my refusal to denounce the military does not mean that I support the centrality of the military in society; rather, it speaks to my desire to recognize the nuances and complexities of servicewomen's and society's relationships with the military—both positive and negative.

Significant changes to military maternity culture are needed, and this book argues, echoing other feminist scholars, that to rectify the problem and help servicewomen, policies are not enough; the milieu of military culture must be addressed. There is a disconnect between policy and culture, which is why the U.S. military is still struggling when it comes to retaining servicewomen. This is noteworthy, because if an organization so focused on obedience to the rules is not significantly affected by these policy changes, how can we expect other organizations outside the military with less generous policies to see progress?[88] This book is an effort to expose this policy-culture disconnect in the military and open the door for envisioning a different military culture, and, eventually, a different workplace maternity culture in U.S. society.

The first step in moving toward addressing changes in the military is to understand the issues surrounding military maternity as systemic, not individual, problems. What becomes clear throughout the research is that these problems are linked to the military culture, which is rooted in hierarchy and masculinity. In their research on sexual harassment of women in higher education, Johnson et al. make a distinction between organizational *climate* and *culture* that is relevant to this study. As they explain, organizational climate "plays a primary role in facilitating" problematic systemic behaviors, in this case, discrimination against pregnant servicemembers. They explain that organizational climate is directly linked to an organization's policies, and define it as "the shared perceptions within an organization of the policies, practices, and procedures in place (i.e., why they are in place; how people experience them; how they are implemented; what behaviors in the organization are rewarded, supported, and expected)."[89] Therefore, throughout this book when I examine the policies and procedures in the military related to maternity, and the ways that servicewomen report experiencing and responding to them, I am examining the military's organizational climate. As it becomes clear, just because policies are in place does not mean that the behaviors supported by the policies are actually rewarded. This is because the military's organizational *culture*—or the beliefs, assumptions, and values that are held collectively by the members of the military—are at times in tension with the policies. Climate reflects the culture, and the culture guides the climate, and in the case of the U.S. military, it becomes clear that the hypermasculine, hierarchical, and patriarchal culture of the military influences the perceptions of policies, including new policies related to maternity. For this reason, Johnson et al. argue that climate and culture must be addressed together, because conflict between them will result in a failed attempt to change.

Second, I argue that to address change, the voices of the stakeholders must be present. As I noted previously, including the voices of those most affected by these policies—the servicewomen—is an important aspect of my method. This inclusion is heavily influenced by my critical feminist orientation to research. Without including the stakeholders in the conversation, effective change will be much more difficult. Johnson et al. also advocated for this in their research on sexual harassment, arguing that researchers and policy makers must "move beyond legal compliance to address culture and climate" and instead "engage and listen to" those who are most affected by the cultural and systemic problems in place. Oftentimes those most affected by a problem also have thought through potential solutions, but they are afraid, or have no outlet available, to voice their opinions, suggestions, and experiences.

Finally, following Ivie, I suggest that we also shift our approach to "thinking about social problems as rhetorical problems and about potential correctives as rhetorical correctives."[90] For example, as I have explained, and as I will continue to reiterate, there is a very circumscribed notion of what it means to be a servicemember in the U.S. military. From a rhetorical perspective, we can ask how to constitute the identity of a servicemember differently, and how changing that point of view can influence thoughts, actions, and interactions. Doing this is what Fixmer-Oraiz refers to as investing "in the radical possibilities of rhetorical (re)invention," challenging the status quo, and looking to new possibilities that reflect the current needs of those serving in the U.S. military.[91] This means that the conversation is larger than and transcends policies, and instead looks to ways that a responsive mechanism could be put in place, during servicewomen's maternity experiences and beyond, in order to address the current issues.

This book is organized in a way that follows the continuum mentioned by Michelle earlier—pre-pregnancy, pregnancy, and post-pregnancy—and is written with the rhetorical mindset advocated by Ivie, Fixmer-Oraiz, and others. It also reflects the words of Carol Burke, who studied military folk culture and argued that "cultures are not determined, nor do they determine. On the contrary, a culture is a made thing or a set of practices subject to change."[92] Indeed, change is possible, and in a military environment that is undergoing significant demographic changes, it is time to step outside of the deterministic mindset that has led the military thus far. This shift can have significant effects on the ways people craft, enact, and respond to policies, and may ultimately change the military maternity culture.

2 Contextualizing Military Maternity Experiences

> I've been in combat. . . . See, a lot of people don't realize this. We've been front line for years. This entire war.
>
> —Magellan

In 1970, unmarried Navy sailor Anna Flores became pregnant. Flores miscarried before she and her fiancé, who was also an enlisted sailor in the Navy, could get married. Yet despite no longer being pregnant, her commanding officer wanted her discharged based on Navy regulations at the time, and recommended, "In spite of FLORES [*sic*] excellent professional performance and her strong desire to remain in the Navy, retention is not recommended. To do otherwise would imply that unwed pregnancy is condoned and would eventually result in a dilution of the moral standards set for women in the Navy."[1] By referring to "moral standards set for *women* in the Navy," this statement points to a discriminatory military culture that set different moral standards for women and men. Because there were no standards for unwed fatherhood in the Navy, the military in the 1970s was perpetuating the antiquated nineteenth-century belief that women should be held to higher moral standards than men.[2]

Citing the biased moral standards, Flores filed suit before the U.S. District Court in Pensacola, Florida, to stop the Navy from discharging her, contending that "the Navy did not apply to men and women a single moral standard in determining retention in the service, so that her severance from service on that ground and the recommendation was unjustifiable discrimination violating the equal protection standard of the due process clause of the Fifth Amendment to the Constitution of the United States."[3] Ultimately, Flores argued that she experienced unconstitutional discrimination leveled against women who became pregnant and were discharged, while the men involved suffered no discipline. At the time of *Flores v. Secretary of Defense*, the deputy chief of naval personnel, Admiral Plate, testified that he did not agree with a single standard of morality for men and women. In fact, he argued that if there was a single moral standard, it would enable men who were looking to find a way to avoid their obligation to service "to find women willing to assist them in achieving violations of the morality standard to which military women were already being held."[4] Plate's statement is problematic for at least three reasons. First, it confirms that there were no moral criteria for men, therefore emphasizing a double standard. Second, it places blame on women who would potentially "assist" men in violating moral standards. Third, it shows how the belief that pregnancy is often used as a means to avoid military obligations has existed at least since women were integrated into the armed forces. This, of course, flies in the face of a history of women fighting for the right to serve in the military. In Flores's case, her commander said she exhibited a "strong desire to remain in the Navy," yet she was denied that opportunity because she violated moral standards for female servicemembers.

Furthermore, the *Flores* case emphasizes the understanding that pregnancy is the sole responsibility of women. This type of rhetoric perpetuates the ideology of responsibilization by rendering the men involved invisible and relieving systemic factors of any responsibility. In Flores's case, her fiancé was allowed to stay in the armed forces despite his involvement in the pregnancy. Because the unique structure of the military requires servicewomen to report their pregnancies so quickly (so that plans for replacements can be put in motion), it is likely that at a different place of employment, Flores's supervisors may not have even known she was pregnant before she miscarried, and therefore could not have discriminated against her. Flores's story is part of a long history of women fighting for the opportunity to serve in the U.S. armed forces, but being denied or facing barriers due to their sex and gender. Many of these discriminatory barriers continue to affect servicewomen today, and contribute to the policy/culture disconnect that makes maternity policies less effective.

WOMEN AS MORALLY SUPERIOR

Women have historically been defined as different from men, and one of the most prominent ways this has been reinforced is via the public and private spheres and their association with gender.[5] For example, because men have often been the ones who have worked, they have traditionally been associated with the public sphere, whereas women have been associated with the private, domestic, child-rearing sphere. The two spheres have served to rhetorically and materially keep men and women separated. Therefore, an aspect of the private/public dichotomy is that in the private sphere, removed from the politics of the day, women were presumed to be morally superior and pure.[6] As many are aware, this moral superiority was one of the main arguments against women's suffrage and was also used as a reason to keep women from joining the military—why corrupt the morally superior sex through participation in men's not-so-moral activities? This ideology was often used as an argument to discriminate against women, as was noted in Flores's situation, and was a foundational aspect of many of the initial service opportunities created for women.

For example, because the Women's Army Auxiliary Corps (WAAC, created in 1941) and Women Accepted for Voluntary Emergency

Service (WAVES, created in 1942) were not part of the *regular* services, separate standards and rules were established for them. The standards for women could be much stricter, because they did not participate in a compulsory draft like men.[7] Therefore, women who served in WAAC or WAVES were "required to be of high moral character and technical competence."[8]

Although WAAC, WAVES, and the Flores case are in the past, it can be argued that women are still held to higher moral standards today, especially when it comes to issues related to women's reproductive bodies. For example, Miranda, a Navy officer, explained that in the Navy, there is a stigma for servicewomen to ask for birth control before deployment, because it carries the assumption that the primary reason women are asking for it is to avoid pregnancy when they have sex with a fellow servicemember on deployment, which is prohibited. This ignores the other reasons women use birth control, such as predictable menstrual cycles and menstrual suppression. Yet the Navy will pass out condoms (presumably for male servicemembers) when it pulls into a port.[9] She explained, "Every port does that. It's on the quarterdeck as you get off the ship, everybody has to go through one point to get off the ship and there's this big bin of condoms. Oh, and there are pictures, very graphic pictures of what happens if you don't use condoms." Based on Miranda's description of its condom practices, it seems the Navy assumes men will have sex. Therefore, men are encouraged to use condoms to avoid contracting sexually transmitted infections (STIs), and there is no concern or mention of the fact that men who do not use condoms may impregnate a woman on their port of call (of course, if these women become pregnant, they do not compromise troop readiness). Whereas servicewomen feel stigmatized for asking for birth control because they should not have sex, men get condoms because, even in the present day, they are not held to the same standard.

Indeed, despite the years that have passed since *Flores*, women are still held responsible for sex and resulting pregnancies, while the men involved go unscathed. As military policies continue to allow more women to serve in more roles—with one of the most controversial and extreme being the lift to the ban on women in combat positions in 2015—critics continue to raise the argument that allowing more women into various roles in the military will inevitably detract from the mission because it will lead to sex between servicemembers.[10] What these critics do not recognize, however, is that ultimately, despite the military's general policy for abstinence-only deployments, "women [shoulder] nearly all of the risk and blame when soldiers do decide to have sex on deployment."[11] Furthermore, these views perpetuate problematic understandings of men as unable to control their sexual desires in the company of women, therefore holding women—and not men—responsible for men's actions.

WOMEN AS PROFESSIONALLY INFERIOR

In addition to being considered morally superior, women have often been treated as professionally inferior. Much of this is likely due to the separation of life into the two spheres mentioned earlier—the private and the public—wherein women are assumed to be part of the private domestic sphere and men part of the public, professional sphere. As a result, the prevailing notion of the ideal worker is male-based and male-biased and "presumes a continuous professional life with little pause for private interruption. . . . [A 'universal worker'] exists primarily for work—a disembodied being whose sexuality, emotions, and capacity for procreation remain invisible."[12] Despite its social construction, this belief is so deep-seated that it is often understood as natural/innate. Not surprisingly, the military has reflected these cultural beliefs.

For most of U.S. history, women were not allowed to officially serve in the military. Yet many women have found ways to be engaged in national defense in various roles since the birth of the United States, often serving in auxiliary—and gendered—roles such as nurses, laundresses, and seamstresses.[13] Women who did serve in auxiliary roles were not recognized as members of the military, but as wives of soldiers, reflecting the general legal status of women in the United States at that time. In some instances, women who possessed a desire to serve in the armed forces beyond their traditional supportive roles would disguise themselves as men, but these women were expelled as soon they were discovered.[14]

As time went on, the military started programs that allowed women to serve as nurses and temporary members of the armed forces in times of war. These opportunities were gendered, and did not offer women the chance to serve in the same capacity as their male peers. The Army Nurse Corps Auxiliary was established in 1901. Then, in response to the demands of World War I, in 1917, the Naval Reserves allowed women to enlist and perform clerical duties, with the Marines following suit. Shortly after the Marines' recruitment efforts, however, the Armistice of November 11, 1918, was signed, and women were no longer needed. Therefore, the roles reverted back to what they had been during peacetime, which consisted mainly of the Nurse Corps.[15]

Then, in 1948, the Women's Armed Services Act (WASIA) served as the official integration of women across the board into the *regular* military.[16] Although it was (and still is) hailed as a major step for women in the military, the WASIA in reality "impose[d] and perpetuate[d] a set of legalized institutional discriminatory standards."[17] For example, servicewomen could not achieve ranks of colonel, general, or admiral, and their representation was capped at 2%.[18]

And if a woman had any dependent children, she could no longer serve, as her maternal obligations were deemed incompatible with her military service. Fathers, of course, were allowed to continue serving. Additionally, WASIA authorized the various service secretaries to "terminate the service of a female member, enlisted or commissioned, under regulations established by the President," most prominently by establishing the grounds to separate women from the military on the basis of pregnancy and parenthood.[19] As a result, despite the so-called integration of women into the armed forces, the act itself served as a way to make official the roles women had already been performing—and pay them for their work—rather than actually granting equality and access. It also perpetuated a rhetorical landscape that would allow for the involuntary separation of women and discrimination against women on the basis of sex, or being different from men.

WOMEN AS INNATELY MOTHERS

Women's presumed moral superiority and professional inferiority are closely linked with one of the most prevailing beliefs about women historically and currently (as will be noted further in chapter 5): that women are first and foremost destined to be mothers. Holm elaborated that based on this belief, "a woman's natural responsibilities as a wife/mother were inherently incompatible with her military duties, and that whenever these two came into conflict, the former must take precedence, irrespective of her professional value to the service and often in total disregard for her own desires or best interests."[20] This belief became official military policy in 1951 when President Harry S. Truman signed Executive Order 10240, three years after WASIA integrated women into the military. Truman's order delineated the "regulations governing the separation from the service of certain women" serving in the armed forces.[21] Truman explained that a servicewoman may be "terminated, regardless of rank, grade, or length of service" for reasons that are the same for a man *as well as* when a woman:

(a) is the parent, by birth or adoption, of a child under such minimum age as the Secretary concerned shall determine,
(b) has personal custody of a child under such minimum age,
(c) is the step-parent of a child under such minimum age and the child is within the household of the woman for a period of more than thirty days a year,

(d) is pregnant, or

(e) has, while serving under such commission, warrant, or enlistment, given birth to a living child.

If any of these conditions are met, "such woman may be totally separated from the service by administrative action by termination of commission, termination of appointment, revocation of commission, discharge, or otherwise."[22] As Holm explained, this order was meant to be *permissive*, yet across the board the services chose to treat it as a *mandate*.[23] Under this order, women who had any parental obligations—including those who were stepparents who housed a stepchild approximately 8 percent of the entire year (part c above)—were to be terminated from military service. Clearly, the standards for military service followed the gendered understanding that women (including stepmothers) should be defined by their obligation as the primary caregivers for children and must be home to care for children, while fathers (even when they are the biological/natural fathers) may be absent. It also is a very patronizing policy in which the military made decisions about the servicewomen's own family obligations.

Despite these prevailing cultural beliefs, voices of dissent were present. Some argued that men's personal lives were not regulated as closely as women's, an argument that continues today.[24] Others, such as Rear Admiral Clifford A. Swanson, the chief of the Navy's Bureau of Medicine and Surgery, cited pregnancy as a "normal biological phenomenon" and that "it would appear to this Bureau to be no reason for terminating the service of personnel who are pregnant but physically able to perform their duties."[25] Yet these seemingly radical beliefs about the ability of women to be pregnant, have children, and continue to serve in the armed forces were largely ignored. Instead, cloaked in arguments about the military's "mission" and the need for "readiness," the response was that women who are pregnant or mothers could not and should not serve as members of the U.S. military, and instead should devote themselves to their roles as wives and mothers.[26]

As a result, pregnant women were involuntarily separated as soon as the pregnancy was discovered, like the case of Flores that opened this chapter.[27] This was a difficult situation, because most of the women serving in the armed forces were of childbearing age and therefore more likely to get pregnant, whether intentionally or unintentionally.[28] This also meant that, as opposed to men, if a woman had a child, the military could not be her lifetime profession, because being pregnant and/or a woman with children was deemed incompatible with a military career.

Hays and others have argued that, around this time, a new ideology pertaining to motherhood emerged, called "intensive mothering."[29] Despite the fact that women entered the workforce during World War II like never before (in order to fill the voids left by men who had gone to war), there was simultaneously a growing ideology that insisted that women's priorities should first and foremost be their children. The separation of the public and private spheres and the rise of intensive mothering ideology rhetorically reinforced that women are always already meant to be mothers.[30] The problem, of course, is that this notion of women, as well as the understanding of the public and private divide, creates problems for working mothers. As a result, although women have been making gains in the workplace, the ideologies that existed and influenced Truman's executive order in 1951 continue to make it so that "motherhood still does not easily accommodate highly demanding jobs."[31]

INTEGRATING MATERNAL BODIES IN THE MILITARY

In 1974, shortly after the *Flores* case that opened this chapter, Stephanie Crawford, a female marine, was pregnant out of wedlock. Yet the outcome of her case was dramatically different from that of Flores. At that time, the Marine Corps had a policy that even if a woman gave up all custody and control of her child, she was to be discharged, echoing the sentiments of Flores's commanding officer stated earlier. Additionally, if a woman was discharged for pregnancy, the Marine Corps had a patronizing policy that the woman's parents should be notified of the reasons for her separation, regardless of the servicewoman's age.

Crawford filed suit, and the court found that it was unconstitutional to assume a pregnant marine (or servicemember) was permanently unfit for duty, stating, "Under this analysis the Marine Corps regulation here established an irrebuttable presumption that any pregnant female in the Marine Corps is permanently unfit for duty. Such a presumption constitutes a heavy burden on the exercise of the individual's protected freedoms of personal choice in matters of marriage and family life, freedoms protected by the Due Process clause of the Fourteenth Amendment."[32] This case was important in the long legacy of legislative and policy battles that were fought in order to eliminate the barriers that worked to keep the U.S. military a predominantly male institution.[33] As the United States transitioned to an all-volunteer force after the draft ended in 1973, the U.S. military began to actively recruit women to its ranks, in order to maintain troop numbers.[34] It therefore would have to negotiate the two very challenging issues of pregnancy and parenthood that corresponded with utilizing "the talents of women of childbearing age."[35] Additionally, in June 1974, the secretary of defense ordered the secretaries of military departments to stop involuntary separations from the military due to pregnancy. The policy change was to be implemented by May of 1975.[36]

Despite the *Crawford* victory and the policy changes, the attitude that pregnancy in the military is presumptively problematic has not dissipated. Although women now have a choice to stay or leave when pregnant, some have argued that allowing pregnant servicewomen to stay and making concessions to transfer them out of forward-deployed units jeopardizes not only the combat readiness of the troops but also the career of the pregnant servicewoman.[37] Others contend that pregnancy as well as children are compatible with a military career.[38] As these disagreeing viewpoints continue, additional military policy changes have gone into effect that work to integrate women into the ranks.

Gender-Neutral Uniforms

One of the ways that some understand women to have been viewed as inferior is by servicewomen's different (read: feminine) military uniforms. In 2015, Secretary of the Navy Ray Mabus wanted gender equity to be a priority, and to him, this meant "blur[ring] the distinction between men and women in uniform" by having a "visibly gender neutral Navy."[39] Mabus argued that once the Navy stopped segregating by uniform, it could truly integrate women into the Navy. Therefore, it was announced that female chiefs and officers were to wear the same covers (hats) as their male counterparts, and enlisted females ranked E-6 or below were to start wearing the "Dixie cups."

However, as has historically been the issue when it comes to gender-neutrality, the term *gender-neutral* often actually means "male." Indeed, many feminist scholars have argued that the so-called neutral human is a (white) male.[40] Due to the military's high regard for masculine traits, many female soldiers find serving in the armed forces an uphill battle. As Taber argued, "the way to be a woman in the military is to conform" to militarized masculinity or to become as "masculine" as possible, disguising or hiding any hints of embodied difference.[41] And MacKinnon argued, "to require that one be the same as those who set the standard—those which one is already socially defined as different from—simply means that sex equality is conceptually designed never to be achieved."[42] The achievement of masculinity for female soldiers appears to be an impossible goal, since the (hyper)masculine military culture relentlessly reduces women to their *different* bodies. This rings true in the case of the Navy, as well. Instead of creating truly gender-neutral uniforms, the Navy is requiring women to wear the uniforms that the men have traditionally worn.

Although this push toward a more gender-neutral uniform can be seen as a way to create an equal, "genderblind" military, many servicewomen are not in agreement with the changes. For example, Elizabeth, a retired Naval officer, explained that she saw the movement toward a more gender-neutral uniform as a way of masculinizing women and erasing the "awesome history" behind the women's Naval uniform. Her thoughts are significant, so I am quoting her at length:

> And [the admiral] is like, "Well, in the military we want to be uniform. We want to all look the same." And I respect the admiral's position. And my thing is that . . . part of the strategy for recruiting women in World War II, they hired Fifth Avenue designers to design a uniform that would attract women. It's amazing. And that is the uniform that I wore at commissioning. I mean it was the same goofy little hat and nice jacket with the buttons down on the sleeves. And I loved that uniform because it spoke to so much history for me as a woman, but also as a woman in the Navy. And we had the tiara. The tiara was designed by Fifth Avenues. But my thought is having the different uniform it's still a Navy uniform. No one will look across the room and say you're not in the Navy. And it acknowledges that women can be in the Navy as an equal partner but that we don't have to be the same. They don't have to be a man. And I always tell people—*I didn't join the Navy to have a sex change.* I joined the Navy to serve my country at sea. And so the uniform issue to me is just like the pinnacle of that. And on the one hand I absolutely understand the logic that you want to make things uniform. *But by doing so you're erasing femininity. And it's making things more masculine.* And I just wonder if it helps or it hurts in the end. [emphasis added]

Elizabeth's words echo what many feminist scholars have argued—that "gender-neutral" is often coded language that means the ultimate masculinization of women, not a way to meet in the middle and find a truly new "neutral" standard. Elizabeth is proud of being a *woman* in the Navy and proud of the history behind the uniform, and her fear is that if everything moves toward a gender neutral/male standard, the important contributions and history of women in the military will be lost.

Career Intermission Program

A more recent retention initiative in response to the needs of pregnant and parenting servicewomen is the Career Intermission Program (CIP). During my interview with Clementine, an Air Force officer, in August of 2016, she referred to CIP as "a very special program the military offers as of March first this year, which is kind of like a two-year sabbatical." She had her first child while she was active duty, and then she separated via CIP six months after her daughter was born and was part of the second group of people in the Air Force accepted into the program. She explained that female retention was a reason the Air Force was interested in this program. In fact, according to Navy personnel officials, the CIP originated because they were having "considerable" difficulties retaining servicewomen, and based on multiple retention studies between 2003 and 2008 realized it was due to the "inability to address personal and family needs, especially among female service members."[43] However, Clementine also emphasized that it is not limited to females, and that, in fact, in the first round there were equal participants of males and females. Because the military's "up or out" system (where servicemembers must meet certain requirements in a specific amount of time in order to be promoted and remain in the military) does not allow flexibility in the promotion timeline that may be needed if someone wants to have a baby, care for a sick loved one, or go back to school, the military was seeing many people separate earlier than planned.[44]

Although some branches, like the Army and Air Force, have offered CIP since 2014, the Department of Defense authorized all branches to offer it starting in 2018.[45] Designed to allow servicemembers "the flexibility to manage short-term conflicts between service responsibilities and life priorities," the goal was that the program will help with retention efforts because people who would normally separate early would decide to continue serving.[46] Essentially, the objective was to offer an alternative work/life balance option for servicemembers who were planning to separate. Those who take advantage of

CIP have their promotion clock paused, and they cannot be penalized for taking time off. When they come back to work after their CIP is over, which can range from one to three years, their promotion clock starts back up as if they had never been gone. Part of the service agreement for CIP is that servicemembers will serve two months on active duty for each month of inactivation while on CIP.

Despite the wide availability of the program across the services, and the fact that all services herald it as a "role model for military flexibility," very few people have taken advantage of the opportunity.[47] In the initial years of the program, from 2009 to 2015, the troops who actually signed up and were accepted were less than 10 percent of that allowance.[48] Since 2016, Congress has allowed four hundred servicemembers per branch to participate, but the highest participation to date has come from the Navy in 2017 with thirty-six servicemembers.

Even with the low participation, there were efforts to institutionalize the program, as it was set to expire at the end of 2019. In October 2018, DoD Instruction 1327.07 made the CIP permanent.[49] Some believed that institutionalizing it would help with participation and perhaps assuage the fears that keep people from applying for the program in the first place. Journalist Scott Maucione reported that the military believes there are three main reasons why people are not applying in larger numbers to the program.[50] First, many are not aware that Congress now allows up to four hundred people *per branch* to be in the program each year, thinking that it is much more limited. Second, many servicemembers are wary of the idea that taking time off will not affect their promotion timeline. Instead, many believe that there will be a post-intermission impact on their upward advancement, even if there is not supposed to be. Third, the income while on CIP is very small, making it difficult to provide for oneself. Servicemembers do get to keep medical and dental benefits and get a funded move to the location where they need to be for their CIP, but they only earn 5 percent of their base pay, which can be a significant hardship and/or cost prohibitive in many cases.

What is most interesting about CIP in terms of this book, is the emphasis on gender-neutrality, despite the impetus for the policy being the large numbers of servicewomen separating from service due to work/life balance hardships. As Clementine noted, the military was experiencing a "drain of talented or trained people because females tend to be the ones that, you know, they take care of the family or they're the caregivers. But they had this drain of people who were leaving the Air Force permanently but for things that they considered to be temporary problems." However, whereas going back to school or caring for a sick loved one may, indeed, be "temporary problems," Clementine recognized that, "It's going to be very hard when I have to go back in a couple years, because for me, having children is not a temporary problem."

Even in Clementine's discussion, her words frame pregnancy as problematic—as a "temporary problem." Constructing pregnancy as a "temporary problem" with a temporary fix will not ultimately address the systemic issues involved, as will be demonstrated in the following chapters. The struggle for work/life balance for pregnant and parenting servicewomen is ongoing, especially in this culture that emphasizes "intensive mothering."

Postpartum Policies

Another effect of eliminating the policy to discharge pregnant servicewomen was that servicewomen would now be returning to work after giving birth to a child and want to continue to provide the child with breastmilk via pumping during work. This meant that the military needed to create policies that address this change in military culture. This will be discussed further in chapter 5, so I will only briefly touch on it here.

Robyn Roche-Paull, the author of *Breastfeeding in Combat Boots* and a former servicewoman, explains that when she was in the service in the 1990s, there were no policies regulating breastfeeding or pumping. And because the environment was one in which women's roles were continuing to expand, women were reluctant to push the issue of breastfeeding, despite having "no place to pump, there was no time to pump, there was nothing, plain and simple."[51] She said pushing back at that time felt like reversing the progress that women had made up to that point to be involved in the military.

This is a common tension in feminist arguments, where women want to fight for equality—which often means they feel the need to emphasize their sameness with men, yet they also experience the material reality of their different bodies. Today, breastfeeding policies are much more detailed and comprehensive, and Roche-Paull has created a document that lists all of the maternity leave and breastfeeding policies for servicewomen in all branches of the military.[52] However, as will be discussed later in the book, just because the policies are in place, does not mean that they are effective and/or always followed.

LOOKING TOWARD THE FUTURE

As this brief overview has shown, there are many deep-seated beliefs about women's natural place in society that continue to impact servicewomen's experiences in the military, and particularly those related to maternity. Although not exhaustive, understanding this history will be helpful when reading the following chapters, as it gives a foundation and context for the maternity experiences that will be discussed. Additionally, the military's understandings of gender and sex roles in society are significant because their influence extends to the general public.[53] As Enloe explained, the military's reinforcement of particular beliefs about gender and sex affect "men and women who have nothing to do with the military,"[54] and Brown has further argued that the military "both reflects and shapes socially dominant ideas about gender."[55] What both of these statements point to is the influence military policies and culture have on civilian perceptions of masculinity, femininity, men, and women.

Considering this influence, the following chapters examine the complicated nature of maternity policies in the U.S. armed forces. They illustrate how the U.S. military wants better maternity policies and creates these new policies. Yet, although women in many ways are the same as men, their ability to have babies makes them biologically different from men and they are oftentimes deemed "less than" their male counterparts. Given this reality, we need to affirm that fighting for women's maternity rights in the military by taking women's corporeality into consideration does not undo feminist progress for women's military representation, but rather promotes *feminist progress* for the social and material circumstances facing women today, both inside and outside of the military.

3 Hyperplanning Pregnancies

> There's certainly an impression that women get pregnant to get out of deployment so that's why a lot of us avoid it, you know . . . yes, it creates problems but we also don't want people, you know, we don't want to derail our career but we also don't want people to think that we did it on purpose. Trying to get out of work or trying to get out of deployment or trying to, you know. It's hard enough to be a woman in the military without people thinking that we're trying to get out of doing our jobs.
>
> —Mae

Natalie, an enlisted Navy sailor, had hopes of becoming an officer. An unplanned or poorly timed pregnancy could jeopardize her goal by disrupting the schedule and promotions she needed to maintain in order to meet the qualifying criteria for an enlisted-to-officer program. Therefore, when she and her fiancé, who was also an enlisted sailor, discovered she was pregnant, she thought her plans might have to change. However, Natalie miscarried, and afterward she and her fiancé started taking "all the precautions to not have a baby because deployment was coming up" and she could once again pursue the route to become an officer. Yet, in the months leading up to deployment (approximately a year after her miscarriage), Natalie was pregnant again, and she panicked. Afraid of the reactions she would receive from her command, Natalie decided to secretly receive prenatal care off base. Those providers were not obligated to inform Natalie's chain of command of her pregnancy like Navy medical personnel were (although Natalie was supposed to do so "no later than two weeks" after receiving pregnancy confirmation from her health care provider).[1] She finally told her command in early March, when she was four months pregnant and her ship was scheduled to deploy in twenty days.

After telling her command, Natalie was required to stay on the ship for two more weeks to train her replacement. During this time, she overheard colleagues accusing her of poor pregnancy timing and of trying to get out of deployment. Both of these rumors assumed that Natalie had planned her pregnancy, which she had not. In fact, the belief that servicewomen plan pregnancies to avoid deployment is widespread, and contributed to Natalie's secrecy regarding her own pregnancy. As she explained, "On our ship, they look down on pregnancy, because they think, 'Oh you girls just do it to get off the ship so you don't have to go out to sea, to get out of deployment.' So, they categorize you with that even though *some people* do that, but not everyone." Built in to this assumption is the belief that women can control their fertility and have complete choice over when they do and do not become pregnant. Despite this prevailing belief, a high percentage of women have unplanned pregnancies in the U.S. military: 50 percent higher than rates of unplanned pregnancies in the general public.[2]

As I mentioned in the first chapter, these statistics have likely influenced research on pregnancy in the military that has focused on unplanned pregnancies, with specific attention paid to how these pregnancies affect troop readiness.[3] Multiple studies have found that unplanned pregnancies are more likely to occur among young, single, enlisted servicewomen (often on their first enlistment) compared to officers who were married and had been in the service for an established amount of time.[4] As Holt et al. explained, the discrepancy of unplanned pregnancies between enlisted servicewomen and officers is complex and can be attributed to the combination of a myriad of factors, including age, educational status, marital status, race/ethnicity, rank, and/or socioeconomic status.[5] A 2016 study confirmed that military rates of unintended pregnancies are higher than the national average and discovered that the highest rates of unintended pregnancy were among single active-duty servicewomen.[6]

In addition to demographic factors, at least two other factors may be at play in unplanned military pregnancies: the high rates of rape in the military and lack of access to contraception.[7] Regarding the latter, not all types of contraception are available to every servicewoman, even though the military's insurance covers most types of contraception at no out-of-pocket cost.[8] Even if women are able to access and use contraceptives, women's bodies and pregnancy cannot be fully controlled through the use of contraception; unplanned pregnancies can and do still occur due to the unpredictability of women's "bodily cycles and fluctuating rates of fertility."[9]

Furthermore, many servicewomen do not ask their health providers about contraception out of fear of stigma and punishment.[10] Because the medical personnel are not third-party doctors, but are officers—often male officers who are higher in rank than the servicewomen asking for birth control—it creates an intimidating environment in which to ask for contraceptives.[11] This is because asking for birth control is stigmatized. Miranda, a public affairs officer in the Navy, explained that when she was about twenty-five years old, she wanted to take birth control continuously and not have her period while she was deployed. The doctor would not prescribe it for personal religious reasons. This infuriated Miranda, as it highlighted double standards. She said, "And all I could think on the drive home was, what if I were an eighteen-year-old sailor who had never been on birth control before and here we are advocating that women don't jeopardize their career by having babies while on deployment, and now you're telling me that you hired a doctor that doesn't prescribe birth control?" Additionally, there are different standards for men and women when it comes to birth control. Miranda revealed that in the Navy, if a servicewoman asks "the medical staff for birth control, like a pill or anything like that, then they assume that you're going to have some relationship with a sailor, which is also illegal or frowned upon. So it makes it very challenging for a sailor to have the confidence to ask for that." In chapter 2, I also quoted Miranda explaining how at every port, the Navy supplies buckets of condoms as the sailors leave the ship. In other words, the Navy tells service*women* they cannot have sex while on the ship because they might get pregnant, but it gives out condoms to service*men* with warnings about the sexually transmitted infections (STIs) that might occur if they fail to use protection.

Finally, the Military Abortion Amendment dictates that unplanned and/or unwanted pregnancies cannot be aborted unless the pregnancy endangers the women's life, or is the result of rape or incest.[12] This means that the military's very own abortion policies might contribute to its so-called pregnancy "problem" and limit servicewomen's abilities to hyperplan their pregnancies around the military's schedule.[13]

Given the myriad of factors that contribute to unplanned pregnancies in the U.S. military, researchers have found that servicewomen experience unintended pregnancies at an equal rate while stationed at home base, preparing to deploy, and during deployments.[14] This statistic debunks the belief that there is a relationship between (impending) deployment and pregnancy.[15] Yet the reality is that a pregnant servicewoman cannot be deployed. It is no wonder, then, that despite maternity policies for women that are more progressive than general U.S. society, pregnancy has been, and continues to be, considered one of "the most controversial of all women-related issues debated and researched in the military."[16]

In this chapter, I examine the factors related to pregnancy planning in the U.S. military. Particularly, servicewomen's interviews exposed the contradictions between discourses about pregnancy planning in the U.S. armed forces and the reality of servicewomen's pregnancy planning experiences, once again highlighting the policy/culture disconnect that is so problematic.

PEJORATIVE MESSAGES: STIGMATIZING PREGNANT SERVICEWOMEN

Pregnancies have been viewed as problematic in regard to military service, which is why when women were first allowed to join the armed forces, they were separated if they were pregnant or a parent, as was discussed in the previous chapter. Servicewomen like Flores and Crawford mentioned in chapter 2 fought against this, and eventually women were allowed to continue serving if they were pregnant. Once women were not automatically separated, the number of women serving grew, and as a result, so did the number of pregnancies. In a contradictory twist, the same institution/culture that had kicked women out for being pregnant now circulated discourses that accused women of planning pregnancies in attempts to avoid their duties.

The belief that pregnancies are planned to avoid certain aspects of the job likely took root in the 1980s and 1990s during the Gulf War and the Bosnia intervention when newspapers published demeaning and problematic article titles such as "Pregnancy Kept GI Jill out of War," "A Camouflage Baby Boom?," "Sailor Pregnant to Avoid Tough Duty?," and "70 GIs Leave Bosnia on Stork."[17] Yet, as Holt and colleagues concluded, planned pregnancies "to avoid aspects of military service" have not been supported by research.[18] The interviews for this study confirmed this as well.

Similar to how Natalie reported feeling stigmatized, many interview participants—including Jules, Elsa, Mae, and Jada—used the term *stigma* to discuss the discrimination pregnant servicewomen face because of the widespread belief in the military that pregnancies are planned to avoid deployment and/or physical fitness tests. The term *stigma* originated with the Greeks who used it to "refer to bodily signs designed to expose something unusual and bad about the moral status of the signifier."[19] In the case of pregnant servicewomen in the U.S. military, stigma occurs because servicewomen deviate from the expectations of the ideal servicemember. That is, they do not appropriately discipline their bodies, and/or the "bodily signs" of pregnancy make them different, which is a huge contributor to stigma.[20] As I discussed earlier, research shows that it is *pregnancy itself* that is the (moral) problem. Because there is no perfect time to be a pregnant servicewoman, as will be discussed shortly, whether pregnancies are planned or unplanned ultimately does not matter in terms of stigma. All that matters is that a servicewoman is pregnant. Essentially, pregnant servicewomen inevitably find themselves in a double bind: on the one hand, servicewomen with unplanned pregnancies are accused of poor fertility management and inhibiting troop readiness; on the other, when pregnancies are planned or perceived to be planned, servicewomen are accused of trying to avoid deployment and hindering combat readiness.[21] The comments by Mae, a Naval officer, cited in the epigraph at the beginning of this chapter, explain that many servicewomen consider the stigma when thinking about family planning and also reveal how the stigma adds to the challenges already faced by simply being a woman in the military.

Cindy, an officer who has served twenty years in the Navy, explained that one of the main reasons she found the stigmas so offensive is that they overlooked the responsibility of motherhood as well as how much material change happens to a woman's body after the embodied experience of pregnancy. She explained the "stupid nonsense" assumptions that "people just get knocked up just to have all the time off" are ridiculous. In response, she scoffed, "Are you kidding me? This is an eighteen-year commitment here, people. They don't get what it does to a woman's body, and some women, you know, snap back and some of them—I've still got baby fat, and my baby is ten." The flippant and sexist nature of the stigma frustrated Cindy especially because of how seriously she takes her role as a mother and because of how it has permanently changed her body.

Furthermore, several interview participants believed that the stigma was heavily influenced by the pregnant servicewoman's rank. This is supported by research. For example, Evans and Rosen observed that junior officers and enlisted personnel reported more negative reactions about their so-called "poor pregnancy planning" than those serving at higher ranks, indicating a relationship between rank and repercussions or stigma.[22] Jules, a junior enlisted sailor, confirmed this, and explained that pregnant servicewomen ranked E-5 or below (junior enlisted) are often treated "as if they just graduated from high school" and are irresponsible and making bad choices, regardless of their age or life experience. Jada, a senior enlisted sailor, explained that the stigma existed when she was pregnant with her first child ten years ago and it still exists with her third child, who was two years old at the time of the interview. However, she did not experience discrimination during her most recent pregnancy and attributed it to her higher rank.

Getoya also argued that rank matters when it comes to pregnancy and stigma, specifically when comparing enlisted servicewomen versus officers. She has additional insight because she started her military career as an enlisted sailor and then became an officer. Echoing what much of the research has shown—that the different demographics between enlisted servicewomen and female officers make a difference when it comes to planned and unplanned pregnancies—she stated, "More officers tend to be older, and I'd say the career officers tend to plan their families around their career. There are fewer instances of them getting pregnant so that they can't go out to sea, and I think a lot of that is because our responsibility is greater, and so we choose to do our job over a family a lot of times because we have more people that we're responsible for, whereas there's many enlisted sailors. . . . There are a lot of them, so, yeah, they can be replaced." The interviews for this project also confirmed Getoya's statement. Of the forty-one babies born among all of the officers, seven (17%) were from unplanned pregnancies. For the enlisted servicewomen interviewed, approximately half of the pregnancies were unplanned.

In addition to being accused of trying to avoid deployment, women who had back-to-back pregnancies were criticized for trying to avoid physical training (PT) tests. Emily, a senior enlisted servicewoman, remarked that some service personnel assumed that "if the girl had gained a lot of weight [during pregnancy], they were only getting pregnant again to avoid the body fat test." She explained that if servicemembers are a certain body fat percentage or higher, they automatically fail the PT test.[23] To be sure, many women—including some participants in this study—can and do remain fit throughout pregnancy. PT tests are held regularly and aim to assess servicemember's strength, endurance, and cardiovascular and respiratory fitness. This ensures that members are fit to serve when they are needed. Yet assuming someone has back-to-back pregnancies— which takes a toll on the body and comes with a lifetime of commitments—to avoid work responsibilities is a big assumption.

The stigmas associated with pregnancy in the military carry at least three problematic assumptions. They are grounded in the responsibilization discourse of choice by assuming that all pregnancies are planned to avoid deployment or PT tests. This contradicts many military studies, which found that unplanned pregnancies are much higher in the military than in the general U.S. population, and also ignores the ways that servicewomen's choices are constrained when it comes to fertility planning. This problematically assumes bad intentions on the part of servicewomen. Second, the stigmas rely on antiquated traditional beliefs about gender, such as the belief that women do not *really* desire to fully participate in the organization even though they have chosen to join the all-volunteer armed forces. This view frames women as weak and lazy, unable to handle the physical and mental pressures of the job. This relates to the third assumption that having and caring for children is less demanding work than deployment or taking a PT test, which further legitimizes the exploitation of women's unpaid labor in the home.[24]

RESPONDING TO STIGMA:
HYPERPLANNING PREGNANCIES

Many women responded to the military stigma surrounding pregnancy by engaging in what I have termed "hyperplanning," or planning their pregnancies for very specific times in their military careers.[25] Hyperplanning in many ways reflects Foucauldian discussions of discipline and punishment, as women are expected to discipline their bodies to have babies at certain times or likely face punishment.[26] It is a complicated phenomenon because pregnant servicewomen engage in and advocate for it, therefore contributing to and perpetuating the double bind. By practicing and reinforcing responsibilization (or the extreme emphasis on individual responsibility), servicewomen become cocreators in the circuit of discipline in which responsibilization is institutionalized, communicated, and performed by systems and individuals in the military.[27] This creates a loop wherein women's performances enact responsibilization—even as they recognize it should be resisted—therefore affirming a problematic ideology and further marginalizing and othering pregnant servicewomen. In this regard, hyperplanning is comprised of micropractices in which servicewomen participate in the dominant cultural norms and discourses that stigmatize their own pregnancies.

Hyperplanning discourses are largely influenced by prominent Western neoliberal assumptions about control. D'Enbeau and Buzzanell explain that "contemporary Western thinking about efficiencies in pregnancy" assumes that "women can control, monitor, and reshape all aspects" of their pregnancies.[28] These assumptions once again place the burden of pregnancy timing on women, with the underlying assumption that all pregnancies are by choice. However, the ways that servicewomen are expected to discipline their bodies do not take into consideration how choices may be constrained by variables such as branch of the military, age, infertility, partner's career, and/or deployment schedule.

The communicative construction of hyperplanning expectations is included in military policies. A document that details policies regarding women's rights during pregnancy and the Navy's expectations regarding pregnancy for those interviewed for this project is called OPNAV 6001.C. Naval servicewomen refer to the document as "the Instructions." Within the document is the following statement:

"Servicemembers (1) Are *expected* to plan a pregnancy and/or adoption in order to successfully balance the demands of family responsibilities and military obligations" (emphasis added).[29] Despite the use of the gender-neutral term "servicemembers," this document is implicitly directed toward women. Many interviewees explained that male commanders are often unfamiliar with the Instructions. Furthermore, the word *expected* reinforces the idea that part of a servicewoman's responsibilities is to appropriately plan timely pregnancies.

According to another organizational document that was available to Navy servicewomen at the time of the interviews, the Navy Office of Women's Policy brochure, "Pregnancy and parenthood are compatible with a naval career. . . . Navy encourages family planning to positively impact fleet manning and readiness, and helps ensure success for servicemembers' families and careers."[30] Despite the overall gender-neutral terms in this statement (e.g., parenthood, servicemembers), because it is in a *women's* policy brochure, it is understood to be directed toward a female audience. Although the brochure leads with a statement that parenthood and pregnancy are compatible with a military career, and uses a positive valence in its language, such as "encourages" and "success," it then implies that pregnancy and/or parenthood could hinder a servicewoman's chances for familial and career success if they happen at a time that does not "positively impact fleet manning and readiness." The implication is that any plans other than those that adhere to Navy schedules could mean familial and career *failure*, which places significant pressure on servicewomen to plan their pregnancies accordingly.

NAVY SEA AND SHORE ROTATIONS

Servicewomen in the Navy—including enlisted servicewomen Samantha, Ariel, Magellan, Natalie, Jules, and Jada; and officers Cindy, Michelle, Elsa, Mae, Sadie, and Getoya—explained that expectations for hyperplanning are the most extreme in this branch, articulating intensified responsibilization among servicewomen. Because sailors have rotations of sea duty and shore duty, the Navy expects that women will plan their pregnancies around shore duty to avoid an interruption to the crew on the ship at sea.[31] The sea-to-shore rotation (also referred to as operational and support rotations, respectively) offers a somewhat predictable schedule for servicemembers. Whereas in other branches, such as the Army or Marines, servicemembers may have back-to-back operational deployments, those in the Navy will typically have sea tours followed by shore tours. The predictable nature of the Navy schedule contributes to expectations that servicewomen will plan their pregnancies according to their deployment schedules. And, although there are no official written documents requiring this, as Elsa explained, "kind of an unwritten assumption is that if a servicewoman wants to get pregnant, then they will plan it around shore duty. Obviously, they could never put that into policy." This expectation results in what scholar Joanne Martin calls "corporate paternalism"—an organization's dictating of the reproductive planning of female workers.[32] The more predictable schedule of Navy deployment brings with it expectations of so-called appropriate family planning.

Prioritizing the Navy's Schedule

One of the ways interview participants responded to the Navy's hyperplanning expectations was by prioritizing the Navy's schedule and planning pregnancies around it. For example, Ariel, a senior enlisted servicewoman, explained, "If you're going to get pregnant, you're supposed to do it on shore duty, and that's what I did." Similarly, Sadie, a Navy officer, planned her pregnancy for when she was an ROTC instructor. She said, "If you wanna have children, the Navy's like, 'This is when you do it.'" Additionally, Claudia, who started as an enlisted servicewoman and then became an officer in the Navy, was emphatic about how she planned her pregnancies for specific times that would not negatively impact her career. In her words, "I absolutely planned every pregnancy and I planned it to be at a moment where I would not take a career hit doing it. I've definitely been an operational seagoing command and I wouldn't have even thought about becoming pregnant there because that would've been awful. That would have been a career killer, and I knew it. And if you make a bad choice, you're going to feel it." Furthermore, Paige, an officer, explained, "So, I was always much more careful. I mean, I used birth control. I made sure that I was not in a position to get pregnant, because it would have been just the wrong time for the Navy and the wrong time for me because of that. I mean, they would have to send me somewhere else. I wouldn't be able to do my job." It is interesting how Paige first notes her pregnancy would be a problem for the Navy and then consequently for her. The needs of the Navy, not her, came first, even in her recollection of the events. Mae, a Navy officer, further explained that she stuck to the sea-to-shore rotation, "We planned that we weren't even going to try; there was not going to be a risk of me getting pregnant until we got on shore duty. Because that really does create a lot of problems if you get pregnant while on sea duty. So, in the Navy's view, I planned my pregnancy at the right time.... It would have been much more complicated if I had been on sea duty when I got pregnant." Similar to Paige's comments, Mae also focused on the needs and timing of the Navy instead of her own.

Furthermore, a common concern raised by officers was the negative impact pregnancy can have on a career due to missed assignments and promotions. Cindy contended that having to be removed from a ship due to pregnancy as an officer would be "very embarrassing . . . definitely could hurt your career." Mae echoed this by saying that, while there is no rule or written policy against becoming pregnant on sea duty, "it can and will tank your career." She explicated that if a woman misses a sea duty because she's pregnant, all that is in the paperwork when she goes up for promotion is that the servicewoman only served on one sea tour, not, "She had a pregnancy." Getoya had a similar attitude to Mae. She was very matter-of-fact about it, explaining, "I had to plan my family around my career. I had to plan to grow my family while I was on shore duty. If I was at sea or seagoing command and got pregnant, I wouldn't be able to stay there, and they would've kicked me to shore, and I would've fallen down in the ranks and not been able to stay up with my peers. That's how it is." For her, like Mae, she willingly joined the military—restrictions and all—and therefore she had no one to blame but herself when it came to timing pregnancies.

Additionally, despite having a sea-to-shore rotation, the type of job makes a difference when trying to plan a pregnancy. For example, Elsa, a Navy aviator, explained that for female pilots, there are many more career pressures than there are for public affairs officers. Mae and Elsa explained that the reason for this is because pilots have to continue to fly during shore duty, because of the need to continue to log flight hours. Whereas many women in the Navy can plan their pregnancies during a shore duty and there is no change in their records, Claudia, a Navy officer, explained that it is more difficult to "hide in your record that you were pregnant" as a pilot because there is a very specific career path with specific requirements for aviators in order to promote. Elsa confirmed this, explaining, "As long as you follow that career path, you should stay competitive, but if you go off that career path, you pretty much have no chance." Discussing the less flexible career path for aviators, Claudia explained, "In aviation there is a set career path, like a very set one that you will do this and then this and then this, and if you veer off from that, you've ruined your chances for command. As a Naval officer, command is kind of what you're striving for. So, if you veer off of that path by having a baby, especially for aviators who are unable to fly, then they will not be on the path if they're pregnant." Elsa further described how hard it would be to hyperplan a pregnancy: "The hours, I mean you have a flight schedule and the hours are whatever's on the flight schedule that day, you can't plan anything." Therefore, although the military encourages timing births around careers, for some career lines, it is nearly impossible to do so.

Another reason why family planning is so difficult in the aviation community is because of the training and tour schedules. Elsa contended that "it's very hard to plan, to have a family and have an aviation career as a female" because there are very few windows of opportunity to have kids, and if one is not ready and/or married at that point, they have to wait four more years before they can try again. By her guess, most women in aviation are around thirty-seven years old before they can start trying to have a baby (medically speaking, "advanced maternal age" is thirty-five and is considered "high risk"). As a result, Elsa said that she looked at her situation from a practical standpoint, and did not get to a point where she felt, "Yes, I'm ready now for kids," but instead when it was "good timing" in her career to have kids.

Interestingly, the concern for careers does not just reside in the servicewomen themselves. Clementine recalled telling her commander she was pregnant, and her commander's first reaction was, "Oh my gosh. What's this going to do for your career? What about your upgrade?" She responded with, "Well, I'm not about to forgo the pregnancy just because of an upgrade." She said that her commander caught himself, realizing that his initial reaction was inappropriate. She believed his response was due to the fact that her commander was used to working with men whose wives are pregnant and therefore do not experience the "same physiological changes" and job restrictions that servicewomen do.

Emphasizing Women's Responsibility

Second, many servicewomen responded to hyperplanning expectations by emphasizing women's responsibility and using the rhetoric of responsibilization when discussing their pregnancy planning. Magellan, an enlisted servicewoman, explained the expectation that women arrange to have their pregnancies during shore leave, stating, "You are supposed to plan your children on shore rotation because when you are on sea duty you know you have, um, a mission to protect the country. You are on the go. You are able to get deployed. *And it would be the responsible thing to plan your pregnancy around the sea-to-shore rotation* [emphasis added]. So that's another thing that us girls in the military have to deal with." According to Magellan, it is service-*women*, and servicewomen alone, who must make sure their fertility conforms to military schedules. When they do not, they experience a form of victim-blaming rooted in ideologies of intensified responsibilization. This type of individually focused responsibility once again frames pregnancy as a "woman's problem."

Whereas many of the enlisted servicewomen, like Magellan, tried to hyperplan their pregnancies to avoid punishment and/or stigma, many of the officers cited responsibility and guilt as the main driving forces behind their desire to hyperplan their pregnancies around sea-to-shore rotations. For example, Claudia said, "I purposely had my first child before I was commissioned [as an officer]." This was because her job was such that it would not be wise to have a child for three more years. If she had a pregnancy during that time, she said, "it's just unprofessional."

Michelle described how the responsibility and guilt goes beyond what the policies say, and is part of the everyday culture. She explained, "Oh, it's more that the official channels maybe tell you, 'This is inconvenient, bad for your career, but go ahead and do what you want.' [But] Your peers are telling you, 'What the fuck, man? I am pulling your watches because you are not here and that's bullshit. I got enough work to do, I do not need to be doing your work.' I mean your peers will be very blunt." As Michelle explained, although the policies *say* that they are suggestions, and grant women the ability to do what they want, often it is the servicewomen's colleagues who put pressure on them to make sure the timing of the pregnancies is convenient for everyone, illuminating the policy/culture disconnect.

In contrast, Mae framed the need to hyperplan less as something imposed by the military or colleagues and more as something that the servicewomen voluntarily chose when they joined the military. As she articulated,

And yes, in some ways it's not fair, but we also knew that when we signed up for it. None of us were drafted, so, you know, I knew when I walked into it that . . . some of my family planning was gonna revolve around what the Navy wanted. . . . I think in a lot of ways we have moved past men/women—like we need bodies who are qualified and can do the job. And it just happens that a pregnant woman can't . . . there's plenty you can do on shore duty but, you know, what we need is people who can be on ships.

In Mae's mind, then, the policies and reality are not sexist and promoting a binary of men versus women as much as they are practical.

Voicing Frustration

Finally, although many were able to adhere to the Navy's expectations to hyperplan and did not seem to have a problem with it, others voiced frustration with the written and unwritten standards. Roxanne, a Navy officer, had unique circumstances with multiple variables, which included the timing of when she met her husband, her own age, her sea-to-shore rotations, and the fact that she had to use in vitro fertilization (IVF). In her words,

The one thing I have been told many times is, "You can have your baby on your shore tour." Which—I'm sure you know, every three years your ships go sea to shore, sea to shore. *Oh, I'm sorry, I actually didn't meet my husband until the end of my shore tour. So, I'm sorry, I didn't plan that so well for the military. Next time, I'll be more careful, and make sure I meet him earlier.* It's frustrating, 'cause I'm on my shore tour. You don't think I'm trying to date and trying to find the one I'm supposed to be with, like really? Like, I'm just supposed to plan my life that way. I didn't find him. I didn't know I was going to get married. And then it turns out, on my sea tour, I'm thirty-three years old, you're hitting high risk at thirty-five, my husband's forty-two. He doesn't want to have a baby very old. So, it's like I couldn't just wait a couple years. Plus, me doing IVF, specifically, I didn't know if it was going to work the first time. Maybe it would have taken me two or three times. So, each time you do IVF, you have to wait six months to try it again.

So, it's like, well, I had to start as early as possible, because I didn't know how many years I was going to be doing this. *So, the thing I had heard the most of is, you should plan it for your shore tour, which I just think is hilarious, because you can't plan life like that.* It happens, the time presents itself, and sure that would be the best option if you have the ability to wait, great. *I'm sure every person would like to try to make it happen on the best time possible. But it's not always possible to do that. Because for me, I didn't know my husband until I was about to leave my shore tour* [emphasis added].

Roxanne's thoughts raise important aspects about the implicit assumptions hyperplanning contains, including the assumption that servicewomen already are married and/or know the partner with whom they would like to have children, that servicewomen will be ready for children when they are on shore duty, and that age is not a factor when it comes to pregnancy.[33]

Jada, an enlisted servicewoman, also voiced dissatisfaction with the stigma the military associates with pregnancies that are seemingly ill-timed. As she recalled, she became pregnant with her first child while she was on sea duty, which she said was a major "no-no." Eighteen months later, she had her second child, and was moving to shore duty, "so it wasn't the same type of stigmatism that's associated with getting pregnant while aboard a ship." Fortunately for Jada, the timing of her second pregnancy was much more "acceptable" because it did not interfere with the military's schedule.

To conclude, hyperplanning is complex, and it is often closely related to biology and gendered expectations. Sadie discussed the different standards for women and men due to women's biology. She recalled overhearing her fellow junior officers (JOs) talking about a pregnant instructor pilot who was on shore duty. The other JOs were saying "how it's so messed up that she got pregnant because she was at a good shore tour assignment for hard chargers, people that wanna, you know, do well and stuff. . . . Saying basically a woman can't have children and be a successful officer." The comments by the JOs are problematic for many reasons. The instructor pilot's pregnancy was well timed (during her shore duty), yet she was still stigmatized. This contradicts the information in the policies and the unwritten rules the servicewomen discussed earlier about having babies on shore duty to avoid stigma. It shows that what seems to be a simple and straightforward guideline really is much more complex. Furthermore, as Sadie explained, there was the assumption that, although men can have children and have successful careers as officers, women cannot. Finally, the rhetoric of choice is present, which once again places the onus on servicewomen, and gives them a sense of agency, even though much of the time the so-called choices are constrained and/or made within very limited parameters.

WHEN HYPERPLANNING FAILS

As I mentioned earlier, corporate paternalism's advocacy of hyperplanning situates the needs of military/career above those of servicewomen/personal life, reinforcing that fertility planning should not interfere with troop readiness. It also treats women's bodies as docile machines, which can be disciplined to become pregnant when it is deemed appropriate. Because the mission is the most important aspect of the military, and readiness is a significant component of achieving the mission, planning a pregnancy is important to ensure the troops are ready when needed.[34] Despite best efforts, meeting hyperplanning expectations for pregnancy is not always possible. In the interviews, it became evident that hyperplanning can fail for at least two reasons: a medical failure in terms of birth control, and/ or a change in the schedule around which the servicewomen have planned their pregnancies.

Birth Control Failures

The messages of hyperplanning required by the military can be frustrating, because many times, even with the best planning, unplanned pregnancies occur. Whereas many of the servicewomen interviewed were able to plan their pregnancies, such as Claudia, who stated that she "absolutely planned every pregnancy," and Frida, who had her IUD removed after she was told she would be at a less stressful job for one more year (and was able to have another baby while she was posted there), others were not as fortunate.

Although many are surprised to learn when contraceptive methods fail, approximately half of the women who experience an unintended pregnancy in the United States each year are using birth control.[35] Cindy, an officer, who was able to plan both her pregnancies, acknowledged this possibility, stating, "Not that you can always plan when you have your children, and sometimes, even the best laid plans . . . I mean, you would like to, ideally, have them when you're on shore duty, but it doesn't always happen that way. And sometimes, even if you are having protection, it just happens." In the case of this research, five participants—Natalie, Paige, Alexa, Clementine, and Elizabeth—experienced pregnancies despite using various forms of birth control.

For example, Navy officer Paige's first and fourth pregnancies were both unplanned, although she was able to hyperplan the second in the exact time window—August or September—that she needed to have the baby in order to then go to her next assignment overseas. She said that the fourth baby was "totally unexpected" and made "absolutely no sense" that she was pregnant. She half-jokingly said, "Maybe I just ovulate whenever I have sex. . . . No, my fourth one wasn't planned. Of course not. Nobody has four children. Especially in the Navy!"

Similarly, Alexa, an Air Force officer, was very surprised to find out she was pregnant, since she had an IUD, the contraceptive with the lowest failure rates. Because she was going to be stationed in Italy, she "purposely planned not to have a baby because I knew that would be tough. . . . If I could've planned that one, I would've waited." Clementine, who is a helicopter pilot married to another pilot, was using birth control when she found out she was pregnant.

The pregnancy was a significant change for them, since they were not planning to have any children due to the nature of their careers and the demanding schedules for pilots mentioned previously.

Finally, Elizabeth, a public affairs officer in the Navy, was using birth control when she unexpectedly discovered she was pregnant with her second child. She was on the transition team for the new chief of operations and was extremely tired. She remembers telling a mentor that she had not felt this tired since she was pregnant. Her mentor encouraged her to take a pregnancy test, even though Elizabeth had been using birth control. Sure enough, the test came back positive, and Elizabeth informed her husband, "We have had a failure of birth control."

Some of these failures may be due to what Duke and Ames call women's "fluctuating rates of fertility."[36] This was the experience of Kristen, an officer in the Navy. Kristen and her husband had tried to plan her pregnancies, but after three miscarriages and multiple failed attempts at intrauterine insemination (IUI), she was told by her doctors that she could not get pregnant. She had accepted this reality and was stationed in Guam. Shortly after arriving in Guam, however, she found out that she was pregnant again, and this time her pregnancy went full term, and she gave birth to the baby in Guam.

Kristen's story, as well as the others in this section, fly in the face of pregnancy as a choice. Yet the belief that pregnancies can easily be planned persists and is constantly perpetuated. Duke and Ames argued that despite all of the disciplining, regulating, and controlling by the military, "the implied docility of this arrangement in the current context—whereby the military conditions soldiers and sailors through discipline, training, and occupational socialization to be in a perpetual state of 'readiness'—is compromised by the decidedly indocile nature of women's bodies."[37] In an organization focused on control, this unpredictability is problematic and threatening. Furthermore, lack of acknowledgment of the potential unplanned pregnancies in military policies and by military members can place unrealistic expectations and tremendous stress on servicewomen.

Changes in the Military Schedule

Many of the officers interviewed also discussed how they hyperplanned their pregnancies for the ideal time in their careers—such as, shore duty and/or location—and then the military changed their orders at the last minute. This was extremely frustrating, since the servicewomen had gone to great lengths to hyperplan the timing of their pregnancies and follow both written and unwritten expectations in terms of family planning.

For example, Michelle had just finished two years of sea duty and had planned her pregnancy to coincide with her shore duty. She was an O-5 at the time, a senior-level officer, and was working with a SEAL team. Despite just finishing sea duty, she was receiving significant pressure to deploy. She stood her ground and resisted, arguing, "This is my baby time, I'm having my babies, that's what you told me—that's what Big Navy said is okay, so why are you having a problem with this?" She said that even though she abided by the military's timeline, it still likely impacted her career. This is significant, because despite following the general guidelines—both written and unwritten—and her rank as a senior officer in the military, Michelle's story shows how servicewomen's careers can still suffer with a well-timed pregnancy.

In Tanya's case, the timing of her pregnancy was crucial, since both she and her husband were on active duty and had different deployment schedules. For her first pregnancy, she was coming to the end of her deployment before going to shore duty. There was going to be a small seven-week window of time between when she returned from deployment and when her husband would be deployed, so she and her husband wanted to try to conceive, since it was "the right time" in her career. She explained how she had served many years in the military and had done much planning and waiting for the perfect opportunity, and it finally came. She was her ship's operations officer, so she knew the schedule, and knew that if she was able to conceive when she was home, she would have her baby in September, which would work well with her sea duty ending the February before she would deliver. In order to be proactive, she recalled having "weird, awkward conversations" with her executive officer (XO) and commanding officer (CO) to make sure everyone was on the same page. She said to them,

> Hey look, we may never have this awkward conversation ever again, or we may be having it in another few months, but I need to let you know that when I get home, [my husband] and I are going to try and start our family. We've never tried before. We've never had an opportunity that works with our careers, and so I have no idea how it's going to go, but I'm not wasting any more time.... So, I'm giving you the courtesy of the conversation. My big reason for telling you is I know the ship's schedule. I know we're going in the yards. I want to finish my time here. I don't want to leave early.

Tanya arrived home a few days before Christmas and found out she was pregnant in January. However, the person who was supposed to relieve her could not make it in February, as planned. Her relief was pushed to June, then July, and then September, when her baby was due. The ship would be leaving the yards in July, and she thought, "Well, this is unmanageable now." She talked it over with her XO and CO, because she had to be transferred. When she saw the email come through about her situation, her XO had labeled her "an unplanned pregnancy loss." As a hard-working, hyperplanning servicemember, she was livid. As she explained, "Here I had done all this time and all this planning and all this waiting for kind of the perfect opportunity and had this weird, awkward conversation with my XO and my CO, and they label me as an unplanned pregnancy loss. I mean, professionally, I was devastated." Even with all of her planning and being up front and abiding by the military's policies and recommendations, she still ended up with an inconveniently timed pregnancy by military standards that was labeled "unplanned" despite all of her efforts to plan.

Oftentimes in these situations, the servicewomen also experienced constrained choices when it came to pregnancy timing and location. For example, Elizabeth explained that despite planning for her pregnancy, she ended up with a detailer who "didn't give a shit" even though "he was in charge of our lives and where we were going to be assigned." At eight months pregnant, her detailer offered her an ultimatum: transfer immediately to a job in Hawaii that she wanted, or stay where she was and have the baby and transfer six months later to an aircraft carrier set to deploy that year. She was frustrated, but ultimately did not feel she had a choice, since she did not want to deploy months after her baby was born. She also did not put up too much of a fight, because she did not see it as that atypical for the military, and figured, "I'm not the only one that's getting screwed by the system." So, in the end, she "chose" to move to Hawaii at eight months pregnant. When she arrived, she did not know any of her neighbors, her furniture had not arrived, and the first time she met her obstetrician was when he was delivering her baby. She says she still does not understand why they could not have waited three months to send her to Hawaii. In this case, it almost seems that pregnancy was treated "as punishment for assumed immoral or irresponsible behavior."[38] In Elizabeth's case, and the cases of many of the servicewomen in this study, pregnancy, even if it is hyperplanned and well timed, is still seen as irresponsible if one is to be an "ideal" servicemember.

In another instance of constrained choice, Frida, who was trying to plan her pregnancies around her deployments, tried to deploy between her third and fourth children's births. However, the military would not deploy her because nothing was available for her rank. Then, as she was on maternity leave in July, breastfeeding her seven-week-old baby, her fourth child, she received a call from her chief of staff asking her to deploy in September for seven months to a non-warzone. He apologized for the timing but knew that she needed to deploy to stay on schedule for promotion. Even though OPNAV 6001.C said that "pregnant servicewomen are exempt from . . . deployment until 12 months after delivery," servicewomen can sign a "postpartum deferment waiver" and waive their rights and deploy sooner.[39] Because it was a good location, only seven months, and would meet her deployment requirement, he called Frida on maternity leave, not wanting her to find out about it later and ask him why he did not offer it to her. She was overwhelmed, angry, and dealing with the hormonal changes that happen after the birth of a baby. She said that she tried to get off the phone as quickly as she could because her baby was drowning in her tears as she tried to breastfeed him while receiving the phone call. The deployment would allow her to come back monthly to see her family, but she felt horrible leaving her husband with three kids and an infant who was still breastfeeding. Despite the circumstances, she felt that she needed to take advantage of the offer, and so, given the "choice," she agreed to deploy. Before she was set to deploy, the seven-month deployment turned into a twelve-month deployment.

RESISTING HYPERPLANNING

Although some servicewomen support—or at least, as best they can, adhere to—hyperplanning, others voiced frustration and resistance to this dominant discourse. One way this was done was through questioning the level of control the military has over their family planning decisions, as was the case with Roxanne. Her situation was unique compared to most, because she had to do IVF. This meant that the level of control was even more intense for her than it was for other women. As she explained, the Instructions stated that she had to tell her command about her intention to conceive via IVF.[40] This frustrated her for many reasons, but two really stood out. First, her IVF treatment was not covered by military insurance, yet they still wanted to have control over her reproductive timing. Second, she felt it was very invasive because the "normal everyday woman is not going to tell their boss, 'Hey, I just wanted to let you know I got off birth control, and I'm trying to get pregnant.'" She said that most servicewomen do not tell their command until they are pregnant, yet she had to provide her command with the calendar that stated when she stopped birth control, when she started her injections, when her egg retrieval would be, and so on. As a result, an XO (executive officer) tried to convince her to delay her timeline. She said that this was frustrating, because the Instructions do not say a woman has to ask *permission* but to inform about the intention of starting. As she remarked, "This is my life. You don't tell me when to have sex with my husband, you can't tell me when to have IVF." Natalie expressed similar frustration at the level of control, contending, "We aren't allowed to have babies when we want. Don't tell us wait till you go to shore duty to have a kid. If we want to have a kid now, we can do that." Natalie's words represent her desire to reconstitute what is considered appropriate and inappropriate for fertility planning.

Another way that servicewomen resisted the pressures of hyperplanning was by trying to put their careers in the military into perspective. They had realized that although they often felt guilty about the thought of leaving their jobs during maternity leave, the military does not feel guilty taking women away from their families. For example, Elsa, an officer, described the advice she gives servicewomen thinking about family planning: "I always tell other women in the service that you can't let the Navy run your life if you want kids. Think about it a little bit, but you can only have kids for so long and the Navy or another job will be there." Similarly, Elizabeth said, "But I always said the military will survive. And they aren't going to go out of their way to look out for you." Frida realized the military would be fine without her, saying, "This organization's been cooking along for 242 years all by itself with way better people than me." Candee explained this concept in a bit more detail, trying not to be "too cynical" but instead practical, arguing,

> The beauty of the military is they make carbon cutouts of us for a reason. They put us all through the same training for a reason. It's so that if you fall on the front lines—if you're taken out, in the traditional sense—à la Gettysburg—there's twenty more just like you who have the same training and theoretically the same qualifications. We get put into stressful situations in the military where you're meant to

believe that you're unique and special and you're the only one who can do this, and the reality is that's not true. There's other people.

In each of these instances putting things into perspective meant thinking logically (practical) instead of emotionally (guilt).

To be clear, Elsa, Elizabeth, Frida, and Candee were all committed to the military and had chosen to spend their careers there, some of them recently retiring after a lifetime of service. As a result of their long-term service to the military, they were voicing what they thought were important decisions when it came to priorities, based on personal experience and self-reflection. Elizabeth explained that the types of decisions she is advocating—to make choices that work best for servicewomen and not necessarily the military—can be difficult for many servicewomen because they require selfishness, and "most people who join the military aren't comfortable with being selfish. They joined the military, and 90 percent of the time it's not for selfish reasons. And they're taught and they're trained to think about mission above self. And while that's true in many, many cases, there are many cases where the mission doesn't have to come before self. Like I said, the organization will survive." Candee echoed this attitude, arguing that "in the military it was all, 'can do, can do.' Well, you just 'can-do' yourself to death, and you see so many people that can-do themselves into losing their marriage or being too detached from their children because they're so busy can-doing at work. Misplaced priorities are common. I don't think it's ever intentional. I think it's all with the best intentions in mind, but there's plenty of people who overcommit and then realize they've shorted themselves and the rest of their life." Elsa agreed with the importance of not just focusing on a career if a woman wants to have a family, as well. Because there is always another mark, another promotion, servicewomen may find themselves constantly striving to be successful at their jobs, and then "sooner or later, they'll be looking back and thinking, 'Man, maybe I wanted a family,' and you can't always change that later." These servicewomen speak to the importance of work-life balance in an organization where the balance is much more difficult to achieve, due to the military's high level of control.

A second way servicewomen resisted hyperplanning was by taking back control of their career and personal lives through a rhetoric of choice, and accepting full responsibility for those choices. Tanya's comments show the link between hyperplanning and resistance: "Make sure you have a plan. Do what you want when you want *but* make sure the Navy won't be able to impede on it. . . . So as long as you're ready for whatever the reaction or result is when that time comes, then go for it." What is interesting about Tanya's words are that, although she is advocating for servicewomen to gain increased agency in the decision-making surrounding their family planning, she is also implying the Navy/military is still ultimately in charge, since it may be able to "impede" the plans and/or have a negative "reaction."

Some of the women utilized the rhetoric of choice through the selection of their jobs. As Cindy explained, there is a saying, "Choose your rate, choose your fate." It is well-known that certain rates (jobs) are less flexible than others, so it was common to hear of women, such as Cindy, Elizabeth, and Elsa, who specifically chose to be public relations officers because of the flexibility in the job when it came to having children. In fact, even within her job as a public relations officer, Elizabeth said she chose to take jobs that worked better for her family schedule than for her promotion schedule, which made her career advancement more difficult, but made her home life more manageable. Paige also explained, "I made that choice knowing full well . . . and I didn't want to compete for the top job anymore. Because I had made my choice. I'd had children; I'd had more children."

Getoya also used the rhetoric of choice in explaining her decision-making. She remembers when a senior officer (male) sat her down and said, "Getoya, don't ever choose the Navy over your family. After you retire, your shadowbox isn't going to hug you. It's your family that's going to be there." As a result of this advice, she said she "took the risk" to try to get pregnant, and "If my choice to have a family prevents me from having command of the ship then I was like 'So be it. God's will.'"

All of these examples point to how difficult it is for servicewomen to "have it all," a concept that will be discussed in more detail in chapter 5. Ultimately, the comments from servicewomen above reveal that they find that it is very difficult to "have it all" and instead feel themselves being asked to choose either/or, not both/and, when it comes to career and family. For this reason, some women chose to either leave the military or move to the Reserves. Mae explained that she was going to leave the military when her current post concluded for this very reason. Candee and Sadie both left active duty to serve in the Reserves. Both of them explained that they love the military, and they saw this as a way to continue to serve in the military, yet have more control over their personal lives.

MILITARY RESPONSES TO RESISTANCE

Because the attrition rate of women in the armed forces is significant, often due to the desire to find support for a work-life balance, the military is responding in various ways. As was discussed earlier, one of the significant problems pregnant servicewomen face is the career derailment that can happen due to missed work, especially for aviators. Clementine emphasized this, recalling how she realized all the ramifications her (unplanned) pregnancy would have on her aviation career. Because aviation careers are not often compatible with pregnancies for female pilots, the Air Force (and other branches) has recently implemented a Career Intermission Program (CIP), discussed in the previous chapter. Clementine was given two years to be on CIP, and because CIP is a one-time opportunity, she and her husband decided they would not try to prevent a second pregnancy. As a result, she conceived again shortly after the birth of her first child, and her children would be fifteen months apart, allowing her the maximum time on CIP to care for them and adjust to life with children before returning to work full-time on active duty. For Clementine, and others, CIP offers an opportunity to hyperplan that is somewhat more manageable. (However, some may argue that because the military still controls this leave, and because the leave allows women to completely step away from their jobs when starting a family, it is ultimately confirming that being a mother and a servicemember are incompatible.)

Another option that Michelle mentioned was that some branches of the military were paying for women to freeze their eggs. As she explained, women's eggs could be frozen so they could have their babies later in life, perhaps at age forty, "but that comes with another unreasonable expectation as well." Ultimately, although it is a nice option for women to have such an expensive opportunity at no financial cost, it still does not address the gender inequity when it comes to when men and women in the military can have children and the disparity in how it may impact their careers. Men do not experience a stigma, do not have to take time off work, are not expected to hyperplan, do not necessarily feel the same amount of pressure to balance work and life, and do not have to consider waiting until they are forty years old to have children. Servicewomen do experience these pressures and often choose to either leave the military or sacrifice promotions for the sake of their families. In essence, the message is that men can have everything, but women cannot.

CO-CONSTRUCTING CONSTRAINT

To conclude, this chapter examined the persistence of "pregnancy problem" discourse in the U.S. military despite research that finds pregnancy does not significantly affect troop combat readiness. Ultimately, through macro- and micropractices including stigmatizing and expecting hyperplanning, a circuit of discipline is created. In this loop, both the military institution and servicewomen themselves, even women who recognize it should be resisted, perpetuate responsibilization ideologies. Therefore, despite progressive pregnancy policies, a double bind is created for servicewomen wherein pregnancy, whether it is planned or unplanned, is viewed as a problem.

Additionally, although there are increasingly progressive policies regarding maternity in the military, the policies are still biased and invasive. For example, Clarissa explained that she had to report her pregnancy, whether or not she wanted to do so, and Natalie waited as long as possible before she had to report her pregnancy because she knew it would not be received well. These requirements again put servicewomen in a double bind: if they report their pregnancies early, they are often judged for being pregnant, and if they do not report their pregnancies early, they are judged for not reporting *and* for being pregnant. Servicewomen's marginalization occurs in the construction of a biased policy and occurs again in their experience even when they follow the policy.

Third, although the military has pregnancy policies in place, the emphasis on women's individual responsibility for pregnancy, and erasure of the role of men or the military, impedes any progress that may result from such policies. The erasure of men and men's involvement in pregnancy is accomplished through verbiage in military policies and also through the passive voice many servicewomen use to talk about pregnancy. For example, they often said that women "got pregnant," which implies pregnancy just happens (and the men magically disappear). This discourse continues to frame pregnancy as problematic, takes away women's agency, and makes fathers nonexistent. Additionally, discourses of responsibilization erase the military's role in pregnancy—for example, the fact that servicewomen's insurance coverage may not grant them access to contraceptives—ignoring a significant contributing factor to pregnancy.

Fourth, despite placing intense responsibility on servicewomen for their pregnancies—planned and unplanned—many of the military discourses around pregnancies ignore the fact that women *volunteer* to be in the military. Servicewomen made conscious choices to join the military and serve their country, and they fought hard to be able to stay in the military during and after pregnancy. Yet, the stigmas associated with pregnancy imply that pregnant women are looking for a way out, essentially playing "dress-up" until they are ready to leave and become mothers. Instead of rhetoric that focuses on how servicewomen balance their careers and the demands of pregnancy and parenthood, the discourses focus on how disruptive servicewomen's pregnancies are to the military, essentially ignoring the deliberate choice these women made to join the military in the first place.

Instituting progressive pregnancy policies is not enough to change perceptions and experiences of pregnancy planning in an organization such as the U.S. military. Strong cultural beliefs related to the "ideal" and "normal" servicemember still dominate discourses, and servicewomen become co-constructors of these discourses when they hyperplan their pregnancies. In this way, servicewomen contribute to, rather than challenge, the discourses that can often constrain them. This is even evident through the rhetoric of choice utilized by many of the servicewomen as a way to take back control, yet ultimately revealing that they are reinforcing the cultural expectations. Additionally, servicewomen who cannot hyperplan are framed as impeding troop readiness because they do not adhere to notions of the "uniform" and "ideal" servicemember. As a result, pregnancy is reinforced as a problem.

Ultimately, the relentless emphasis on fertility hyperplanning in the U.S. military also reflects, sustains, and speaks to the broader discursive arena in which women's reproductive rights are continually—and increasingly—under assault in the United States.[41] Hence, these circuits of discipline related to hyperplanning likely exist across other institutions that purport to be inclusive, but marginalize and otherize women nonetheless.

4 Performing Macho Maternity

> The kind of woman that's interested in the military is usually not a frou-frou kind of gal. She's like, "Don't treat me differently."
>
> —Cindy

Michelle, a retired Navy intelligence officer, developed mastitis—very painful inflammation and infection of breast tissue that can happen during breastfeeding—with both of her babies. The second time she had it, she immediately knew what it was, and went to the doctor. At the time, she was working with a SEAL team, and the all-male team had their own clinic separate from the rest of the servicemembers. Recalling the situation, Michelle explained,

> Well, part of it is the military provided health care so they're not just my employer, they're my doctor, and I remember after I had the baby, I had mastitis. . . . And I went to the hospital on base but as the SEAL team, you have your own little clinic because the SEALs are always banging themselves up, and so they have SEAL docs, so that's where we're supposed to go because we're working for the SEALs. So I trot over there and I'm like, "Hey, I got mastitis." And they're like, "What's that?" [laughter] And I think it must have been the second time I had it because I remember knowing what it was and what to do, [so I said,] "Just send me over to the hospital, okay?" . . . So just some non-comprehension with the whole issue.

In Michelle's case, because she was experiencing a specific female reproductive health issue, the SEAL doctors were not equipped with the knowledge to help her. Michelle's comments about how the military was not competent when it came to female health care—and specifically pregnancy-related health care—were echoed by many other participants.

At any given time, approximately 9 percent of enlisted women and 5 percent of women officers in the Navy are pregnant.[1] Despite increasing numbers of women joining the Navy and the military in general, and the new policies that have been implemented regarding pregnancy, many servicewomen interviewed also discussed how military discourses surrounding pregnancy framed their pregnancies as problematic. Yet, I also found that some servicewomen engaged in behavior that reinforced these discourses, therefore effectively becoming co-constructors who perpetuated the views of pregnancy as problematic.

MILITARY PREGNANCY DISCOURSES: MEDICALIZATION AND REGULATION

In the interviews, it was common for servicewomen to say that the military treats pregnancy like a medical problem in need of a cure. For example, Jules, an enlisted Navy servicewoman, reflected, "I guess the military, the military treats your pregnancy more like a condition." Because medicine is viewed as a "curing profession" it encourages everyone, including pregnant women, to think of pregnancy as a "condition that deviates from normal health" and needs to be cured, therefore pathologizing it.[2] Pathologizing pregnancy frames pregnancy as "not normal" and as problematic. Yet pregnancy is a normal and expected and routine part of many women's lives. Because it is relatively recently that women have not been discharged from the armed services for pregnancy, it is not surprising that many servicewomen report that pregnancy is treated as a medical problem in the military.

Framing pregnancy as a medical condition situates pregnancy in the realm of science and devalues servicewomen's personal knowledge and experience. This serves a biopolitical function of normalization, which positions pregnancy as a highly regulated and routine medical problem. For example, Gutmann reported that the Army, in attempting to demonstrate its competency and comfort with pregnancy in the late 1990s, explained pregnancy as "no different than appendicitis."[3] However, this view of pregnancy also pathologizes it, and overlooks how pregnancy can be an emotional time for women, whether one is excited or filled with trepidation at the thought of bringing a child into the world. Comparing pregnancy to the inflammation of the appendix frames it as a medical *problem.* Indeed, medicalizing pregnancy allows it to become part of the process of normalization, where pregnancy is "no longer just a bodily experience that is known viscerally," but becomes an objectified disciplinary process.[4]

Much of the reason that pregnancies are medicalized and pathologized is likely due to the way the military is structured. As Candee, a Navy officer, emphasized, "when you're in the military, they are legally responsible for your care and your safety" which is another reason why everything is so closely monitored. Yet, because of the impersonal and medical way that pregnancies are handled, many servicewomen feel that their personal experiences and opinions are ignored.

Additionally, medicalizing pregnancy ignores the short-term and long-term effects of pregnancy. For example, Claudia, an officer, explained, "It's a medical thing. So anyone that breaks a leg or . . . [is] pregnant is considered needing more medical attention than a ship can provide." In Claudia's explanation, pregnancy is treated in a matter-of-fact fashion. However, treating pregnancy as a "condition" or a "medical thing," akin to breaking a leg, is an invalid analogy that ignores the lifetime of changes that result from pregnancy. Whereas for many broken legs, the condition goes away shortly after the cast is removed, pregnancy may include many bodily and hormonal changes such as intense emotions and significant weight gain. Furthermore, if a woman finds out she is pregnant and chooses to have and keep the baby, it is life changing in terms of long-term, day-to-day effects, since the woman will now have a dependent under her care. Thus, the implications of pregnancy are much farther reaching than medicalizing discourses suggest. Such discourses trivialize the experience of childbirth and medicalize it as a *problem*.

The current medicalization of pregnancies goes beyond pregnancy and is rooted in an intense desire to distinguish women from men based on biology, with the ultimate goal of framing women's biology as not only *different from* but *inferior to* men's. As Young argues, in a culture that "implicitly uses this unchanging adult male body as the standard of all health," women's constantly changing reproductive bodies are a threat.[5] Foucault called this focus "a hysterization of women's bodies."[6] Hysteria used to be a disorder diagnosed exclusively in women (with symptoms such as faintness, sexual desire, coughing fits, and convulsions), and some doctors believed it was what made women different from men (although much of the time it was used as a way to promote women's inferiority to men).[7] Foucault argued that *all* women came to be seen in this way (as disorderly and needing help), and as a result, the female body has come to be considered an object of medical knowledge that must be studied and regulated closely. Because it is the center of reproduction, and because all women's bodies were perceived as disorderly and intrinsically laden with pathology, policing women's bodies, and specifically the functions that have to do with sexuality and reproduction, was deemed necessary. In her book, *From Hysteria to Hormones*, Koerber emphasized this belief, explaining that contemporary discourses today regarding hormones preserve past discourses that frame all women as pathological simply because they possess female hormones, and not due to an event such as a pregnancy.[8] Therefore, whereas one may be inclined to think that medicalization of pregnancies is a positive aspect of our modern era based in "science" or "objectivity," in reality it is deeply rooted and enmeshed in a history that pathologizes women for being women, or for not being men.

Third, pathologizing pregnancy conflates the public and the private because of the military's structure. It was common in the interviews for servicewomen to discuss the very regulated nature of the military in general. Enlisted servicewomen Clarissa, Natalie, and Mary described how the whole system around pregnancy is extremely regulated, and Miranda, an officer, contended that privacy is a casualty of such regulation. As was discussed in the previous chapter, the Navy requires that servicewomen inform their chains of command of their pregnancies "no later than two weeks" after receiving confirmation of pregnancy from their health care providers.[9] Most of the time the health care providers that confirm pregnancy are part of what servicewomen call "Medical"—or military-provided health care on base. Servicewomen are to "go to Medical" to have an official pregnancy test that is then recorded in their files and sent to their chains of command. Whereas a civilian may confirm her pregnancy at her doctor's office and still wait to tell her place of employment until she is past her first trimester (thirteen weeks), servicewomen's employers often know about their pregnancies much earlier.

However, as is often the case, rank can impact this process. For example, Mae, an officer in the Navy, explained that rank can influence how private the information about pregnancy stays, because once enlisted servicewomen tell their commands, "that's immediately eight people that are going to know. Like at that point, it's essentially like this is no longer private information." However, because officers are of higher rank, there are fewer people in their chains of command, so fewer people will know. Additionally, she claimed there is a bit more flexibility in when officers have to tell their commands. Either way, however, it is the servicewomen's responsibility to tell their chains of command about their pregnancies, and preferably before the military's medical provider reports it so that they do not appear to be undermining protocol. As enlisted servicewoman Clarissa noted, "I *had* to let my chain of command know, it was my *duty* to do so whether I wanted them to know or not." As these women related, even with the flexibility officers may have, there is much less privacy when it comes to pregnancy as a servicewoman, because it is part of their job to inform their chains of command as soon as possible.

In sum, medicalizing pregnancy devalues servicewomen's experiential knowledge, emphasizes servicewomen's biological differences from men, conflates the public and private aspects of servicewomen's lives, and places personal reproductive decisions in the hands of the military. This perpetuates a problematic biological hierarchy in which women (and their bodies) are viewed as inferior, and women feel they must find ways to fight this predominant viewpoint. This further enables military personnel to hold servicewomen responsible for their work performance during their pregnancies.

PATRONIZED FOR BEING PREGNANT

The pathologizing of pregnancies often created an environment where many servicewomen felt patronized for being pregnant, thus devaluing their personal, embodied, lived experiences. Specifically, this manifested in the interviews in two primary ways: (1) commanding officers making career decisions for servicewomen without their consent or input and (2) framing pregnancy as a disability.

First, it was common for servicewomen to recall how those who ranked higher than them made decisions about servicewomen's jobs that would impact their careers based on assumptions about pregnancy and servicewomen's preferences. Both Michelle and Paige, Navy officers, used the word *paternalistic* to describe their experiences. Michelle recalled planning her familiarization trips for her new command to coincide with the last few months of her pregnancy. She knew, from experience with her first pregnancy, that it would be easier to travel while pregnant than it would be to travel while nursing an infant (because then she would choose to pump breastmilk while traveling and then ship it, which is much more labor intensive). She received pushback for her schedule, because her command thought it would be worse for her to fly while pregnant. She found the situation to be an issue of "'I'm ready and able to do it and my doctor is okay with it so why don't you just let my doctor decide? I'm a competent female, I can make decisions about what needs to happen, I've gone through this before. You have no clue.' . . . So it was paternalistic of them trying to do what's best for me. I'm like, 'You don't know what's best for me.'" As Michelle explains, she felt that because she had talked with her doctor about her situation, and because she was the one experiencing the pregnancy (with knowledge of what happens to her body *after* delivering a baby, e.g., breastfeeding, lack of sleep, etc.), she should be the ultimate authority when it came to what was in her best interest, not her commanding officers.

Similarly, officers Paige and Lynn discussed how each of their leaderships transferred them to jobs that were less prestigious and less helpful for promotions. Paige explained how she discovered midway through her pregnancy that her boss, the admiral, was planning to transfer her to a job that was not as difficult or prestigious. She said, "I was really teed that he had paternalistically felt like, 'Oh, she's having her child. So, she'll want to go to a job that's easier and not so time-consuming and stuff like that.'" Paige pushed back, and was able to transfer about eight months after having her baby, when she should have left that job anyway, instead of the pregnancy forcing her to change jobs and affect the trajectory of her career promotions.

Lynn, an Air Force officer, said that she was moved to a position that was not what she wanted, and was told, "It's because you're going to need more time with your baby." She felt this was "terrible because (a) I didn't ask for that, and (b) it was a very—in my mind it was a very underhanded way of just moving me. Like, 'Get her out of the way. Put her here.'" She said it felt like a punishment, because they moved her from the flight line, which she said is the "pinnacle" for her as an Air Force officer. Instead, she was stuck in a desk job and felt like they were "clipping my wings. It sucks. You're caged." In these instances, the servicewomen's chains of command decided that they knew what was best for the women and also assumed that they knew how the women would want to manage their time after having their babies without ever asking the women themselves. Paige, Lynn, and others experienced frustration as their commands drew from traditional gender scripts that prescribe women to spend more time at home and have easier jobs so that they can stay home with their children. In law firms, this type of treatment has been referred to as the "maternal wall," which is when male partners assume women who return from maternity leave will not want to work as hard as they used to and are therefore given less desirable and promotable positions.[10] Each woman is unique in how she plans to raise her children and maintain work-life balance, so a one-size-fits-all concept of mothering is not effective, especially in an organization like the military, where many of the officers—men *and* women—are extremely career-driven.

What is more, these types of paternalistic and patronizing discourses related to pregnancy in the military contribute to and sustain those that frame pregnancy as a disability. For example, Sydney, an enlisted servicewoman in the Navy, explained that after she reported her pregnancy, she was moved to a less demanding type of job: "They can send a pregnant woman there, they can send a person with a disability there, they can send anyone there." Sydney's explanation shows how pregnancy and disability are often conflated. Additionally, although enlisted Air Force servicewoman Clarissa said, "I was treated fairly normal for being in the military, which I liked, because I wasn't disabled or anything, I was just limited to some of the things I can do," others had more negative experiences. In contrast, officers Lynn, Tanya, and Elsa voiced how such discourses of disability were frustrating, especially because they felt it devalued their work ethic and also influenced the way their colleagues treated them. Tanya expressed that the labeling drove her "berserk" and that she was "seriously mortified when I got labeled as [disabled]" in the paperwork. She responded, "I'm not disabled, I'm pregnant." Elsa said almost the exact same words as Tanya when she was describing how her colleagues were trying to be considerate of her as a pregnant woman. She said, "I personally don't like how people treat me when I'm pregnant—just, you know, they're like, 'Don't pick that up. Don't carry that. Let me get the door.' I know that they're just trying to be considerate but at the same time it's like, 'Okay, I'm pregnant, I'm not disabled.'" Lynn also was frustrated when she was told not to do certain things. She said that people would say, "Oh, you're pregnant, you can't do this. I'm going to do it for you." And she would respond with, "I can still do things." These comments reflect how some have made efforts to challenge the association of pregnancy and disability, arguing that instead of seeing pregnancy as a *dis*ability, it should be perceived as "an additional ability"—women, unlike men, are *able* to bear and birth children.[11]

To be sure, discourses of pregnancy as "disability" are not unique to the military. Many women in the United States are required to take short-term disability leave as their maternity leave. Buzzanell and Ellingson explained that maternity is seen as a "negative medical condition" perpetuated in large part by discourse that classifies maternity leave as disability leave.[12] This, they argued, frames pregnancy as an illness, creates and emphasizes a false dichotomy of disability/abnormal/woman and ability/normal/man, produces many social restrictions and biases against women, and reinforces—rather than displaces—the incompatibility of pregnancy in the workplace. Similarly, Kornfield argued that because pregnancy physically marks the body as different, this difference often leads to "the intertwining of disability discourse and pregnancy discourse" which "simultaneously reinforces ableism and patriarchy."[13]

Although many American women experience the stigmas associated with pregnancy as disability, because of the comprehensive nature of the military organization as an employer and medical care provider, this understanding of pregnancy and postpartum leave is extremely intense for servicewomen. For example, the language used to describe maternity or postpartum leave in military policy also pathologies pregnancy. Both the Instructions and Guide 8 (a guide to managing pregnant servicewomen in the Navy) label maternity leave as "convalescent leave," implying recovery from an illness.[14] The conflation of pregnancy with disability reinforces the assumption that women's bodies inhibit troop readiness and thus pose a problem to the military's ability to function, a perspective that contributes to the stigma surrounding pregnant servicewomen.

PUNISHED WITH THE UNIFORM

Additionally, many servicewomen viewed the maternity uniform as punishment. As was discussed in chapter 2, the military uniforms for women have been controversial since servicewomen have been in the military, because the uniform's goal is to make everyone appear the same—uniform—yet servicewomen's bodies do not always conform to the male standards and dimensions for which the uniform was created. The visual signifier of a growing belly that oftentimes cannot be ignored or hidden serves as a powerful reminder of the biological sex differences between males and females. Often this biologizing of women means that servicewomen must negotiate a nearly nine-month management of the dialectical gaze, in which they have to balance the demands of being a uniformed servicemember and a pregnant woman.[15]

In the late 1970s, as more women joined the all-volunteer armed forces, it became apparent that there was now a need for a military maternity uniform. The military was fielding complaints that servicewomen were undermining "morale by coming to work in their civilian clothing when they outgrew their uniforms," so the military maternity uniform was introduced.[16] The maternity uniforms have remained relatively unchanged since then. When the interview participants talked about these uniforms, which are completely designed for women's pregnant bodies, two main themes emerged—(1) their appearance and (2) their cost—both of which only affect female servicemembers.

In terms of appearance, servicewomen found them unprofessional and disappointing. Getoya, Elizabeth, Alexa, Cindy, Sadie, Joanna, and Jules all described it as a "tent." As Jules explained, "Think of pregnancy clothes in the '80s, '70s, where the shirt is a big tent. That's basically our shirt. It looks exactly the same [as regular uniforms] except it's a tent." In giving a bit more detail, Getoya said, "The white blouses we had to wear are like a triangle" (see figures 4.1). Getoya and Sadie discussed how whereas civilian maternity clothing is often cinched to give some sort of shape, the military maternity uniforms are one size, which means that as soon as servicewomen's regular uniforms do not fit, they have to switch to the maternity uniform.

Servicewomen's disdain for the uniform was much less about vanity or stylishness than about how it distracted from the job at hand and in many ways robbed them of their professionalism. Officers Cindy, Sadie, Getoya, and Alexa explained how the military maternity uniforms in the Navy and the Air Force make servicewomen look much bigger than they actually are, drawing unwanted attention from colleagues. Sadie said that the few times she was able to wear civilian clothes, her colleagues said, "Oh my gosh, you look like a normal pregnant person." As Cindy recalled, the minute a woman wears "the tent," all of a sudden people "start acting weird around you." Elizabeth said that it is difficult to feel professional when wearing "the tent," and Alexa said that "people look at you and don't think of you as a professional. When they see you, they think, 'Oh, that lady's big.'" Elsa expressed that she hated switching to the maternity uniform "because first, it looks ridiculous, and it singles you out as 'I'm pregnant,' even if you're not really showing yet, and it isn't even professional." The design of the regular uniform pants for servicewomen are a higher rise that, Elsa explained, "hits a little higher than normal pants and so it's right around where your belly is getting bigger." As such, they become uncomfortable sooner

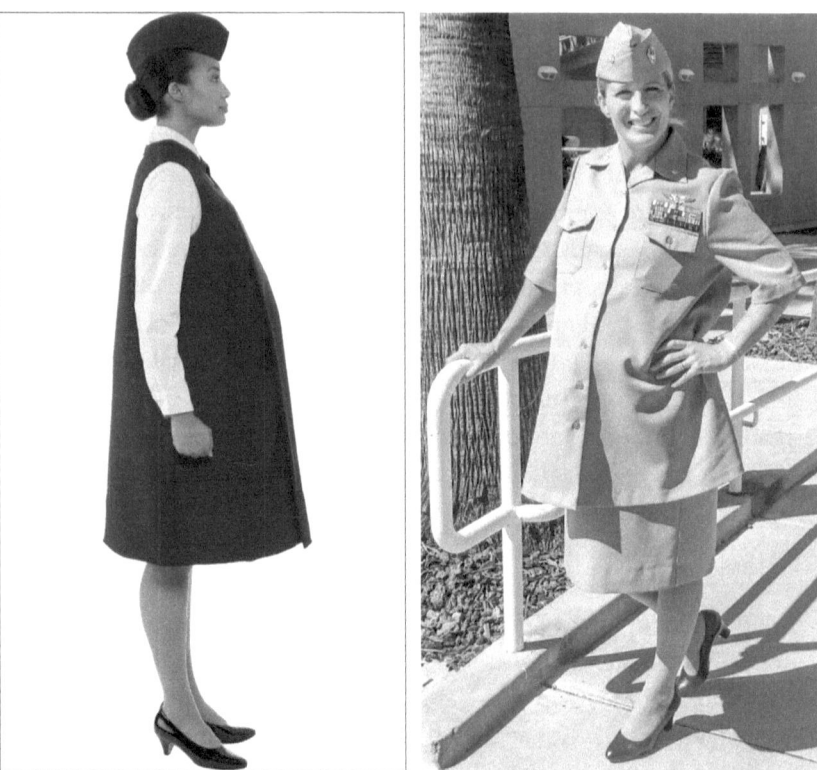

Figure 4.1a Left: Current Air Force maternity jumper. Courtesy of the U.S. Air Force. *Figure 4.1b Right:* CDR Sandy Kosloski, a flight officer, is pictured at seven months pregnant in September 2015 wearing the U.S. Navy service khaki maternity uniform. Photograph taken and provided by her sister, LCDR Colleen Kosloski. Neither of them were interviewed for this project.

than civilian pants might, which causes servicewomen to switch to the maternity uniform sooner than they would normally switch to maternity clothes as civilians. Then suddenly, their identity switches from being a colleague who blended in to being a pregnant woman who stands out as different. As a result, Cindy, Sadie, and Alexa recounted delaying the military maternity uniform as long as they could, which Alexa said was "kind of an unwritten thing that a lot of the officers do."

Second, servicewomen often mentioned how much military maternity uniforms cost. Enlisted servicewomen are given an allowance to purchase two maternity uniforms, but officers have to pay for the uniforms out of pocket. What often emerged around this theme was a discussion of the rhetoric of choice. In one example, Emily, an enlisted Navy servicewoman, explained that her chief forced her to purchase all of the pregnancy uniforms (working, service, service dress white, service dress blue, service dress khaki), even though she really only needed two, and was given an allowance to purchase two. When she told him how much it would cost, she said, "He basically told me, 'You're the one that wanted to get pregnant. Suck it up.'" Similarly, when talking about how officers are responsible for purchasing their own uniforms, Elizabeth said, "Again, the idea is pregnancy is a choice, so you pay for it [the uniform]." Of course, interesting in all of this discourse of choice is the fact that, as was discussed in previous chapters, servicewomen's rates of unplanned pregnancy are higher than civilian rates. As such, this discourse of choice is ignoring the possibility of servicewomen's unplanned pregnancies. Additionally, even if servicewomen do choose to have children, the cost of military maternity uniforms is something that they bear on their own, since their male colleagues who have children (whether by choice or not) do not have to purchase special uniforms. Ultimately, this is another version of punishing servicewomen for being pregnant.[17]

To further complicate the issue of uniforms, the pregnancy uniforms seem to contradict other changes in the military uniform because they make servicewomen stand out due to how unflattering they are and how large they make women appear. Both Elizabeth, an officer, and Jada, an enlisted servicewoman, explained how the military was trying to change to a "gender neutral" uniform, as was discussed in chapter 2. Jada said that women would soon be wearing male covers, in an effort to be "in one accord." Elizabeth said that in the military "we want to be uniform. We want to all look the same." Ironically, at the same time that the military is attempting to make servicewomen more uniform, it is requiring pregnant servicewomen to wear uniforms that highlight them as very different, which could be interpreted as a form of punishment.

POWERLESS IN HEALTH CARE DECISIONS

In addition to feeling patronized and punished when pregnant, many servicewomen cited feelings of powerlessness when it came to health care. To be sure, military insurance benefits are valued by many of the servicewomen. From health care that is covered at 100 percent to only paying for the meals in the hospital when they delivered their babies, many interview participants were very grateful for their military insurance. Yet, as Master Sergeant Mom, an enlisted Air Force servicewoman, explained, "The military does take very good care of you and your family, but again, it comes at a price." Despite how grateful the servicewomen were for the free health care they received, many also voiced frustration and disappointment with their health care when it came to pregnancy. The required reliance on military health care left many servicewomen feeling powerless when it came to making personal health care decisions.

The most often cited complaint among officers and enlisted servicewomen was their lack of control in decision-making when it came to health care providers, in addition to a lack of consistency in the providers they saw for their prenatal care. Although Tanya explained how she had the same midwife for both of her pregnancies, she recognized how unique her experience was. As she said, "Strangely enough, or oddly enough, because it never happens in the Navy, I actually had the same . . . midwife both pregnancies because they [the pregnancies] were so close." It is clear in Tanya's statement that she recognizes how fortunate she was to receive continuity of care, but that the only reason she likely received this care was because her pregnancies were so close together, making it more likely that the same midwife would still be assigned to her and not transferred yet.

In contrast, Roxanne voiced frustration about her lack of control due to the nature of the employer/health provider paradigm in the military. She stated, "Yeah, everything's covered, except they have like this massive control over you." Jules said that all of her civilian friends had much more say in their treatment than she did as a servicemember. For example, she said that civilians have a doctor they see the whole time they are pregnant, whom they can call if they have a question or need help. As a pregnant servicewoman, she said that she got "whoever is available." Alexa explained how "you get assigned" doctors, whether you like them or not. Ivette, an enlisted servicewoman, also was disappointed that there was no consistency in whether she would have the same doctor each time. Instead, she said, "it was whoever's on call." Emily explained that she "did not get the choice of seeing an OB I wanted," but instead had to see whoever was at the Navy hospital, where she also worked.

Furthermore, several servicewomen did not even have the option to see an OB/GYN or midwife—those whose medical training is specifically for prenatal and postpartum care. Paige recounted how she had four pregnancies and never saw an OB for any of her appointments. Moreover, she said she saw a different provider each time. Natalie, an enlisted servicewoman in the Navy, also recalled that her base did not have any OBs, so she just saw a primary care doctor for her prenatal care. As Roxanne, a Navy pilot, explained, "You don't get that continuity of care, or you don't get to really have any kind of say in who you have" as a doctor.

This model of inconsistent providers and/or providers with whom pregnant women are unfamiliar contradicts much research that supports the importance of continuity of care—the same provider or small group of providers chosen by the pregnant woman herself—when it comes to pregnancy.[18] Women who are able to choose their doctors and see the same doctor(s) throughout their pregnancy are more likely to attend prenatal education classes. Additionally, many women who experience continuity of care report better prenatal, birth, and postpartum experiences.

The lack of control in choosing providers was part of a larger complaint servicewomen voiced regarding subpar care. Another issue was that military dependents (e.g., wives of male servicemembers) received better benefits than the servicemembers themselves. Roxanne visited the Tricare insurance offices at the hospital and discovered that if she were a dependent on health care, she would have more agency and freedom than as a servicemember. To her, this was infuriating, especially after she felt she was already making significant sacrifices in terms of her health as a woman. As she described, "I don't see a gynecologist on a yearly basis. I see a flight surgeon. And the flight surgeon does my pap smear, which I'm completely against. And I've always thought that was wrong because they don't do them very often, and they're not the experts, and I don't think that they should be doing breast exams and pap smears because what do they know? They're just a general person, but why do my friends' wives, who are dependents, all get to see an actual gynecologist, who's an expert in the field?" Candee also noted the difference between dependents and servicemembers, because she experienced both firsthand. She explained that with her third child she was still married to an active-duty military member (she had transitioned to the Reserves), and, "It just afforded me greater flexibility and options because I was treated as a civilian spouse. I was a military dependent, but I wasn't beholden to all the active-duty military regulations, which I was in the first two pregnancies." For her first two pregnancies, she had to be seen at a military hospital, but for her third, she had the option to have a midwife and alternative/non-hospital birthing methods. The reality that servicewomen have less of a voice in their own health care than their colleagues' wives do frustrates them, especially since they are risking their lives to serve their country. In response to this and the employer/health provider paradigm, Roxanne remarked, "So if you own our bodies, don't you think you should give us the best care possible?"

The military may respond by stating that it is giving the best care possible—if the military is accountable for the care, they want to make sure it is at one of their approved facilities with their approved providers. Yet, because the military is responsible for the health care of its members and provides mostly free health care to them, there are firm restrictions on the care provided. For this reason, the policy states that servicewomen are not allowed to deliver at a hospital of their choice: "Service members are not authorized to take leave to travel outside their area of residence for the sole purpose of giving birth at a civilian hospital or to deliver or receive other OB care at a location outside of the MTF [military treatment facility] area of responsibility or away from the network provider or TRICARE authorized provider while in a leave status."[19] One consequence of this policy is that the military hierarchy exists in the doctor's office, and the labor and delivery rooms, as well.

For Jules, this was a good thing. She appreciated that she had military providers when she was in labor because "they were able to get in my face and calm me down and get me to focus on things. But I had a lieutenant and a lieutenant commander with me, and I remember the anesthesiologist was the one who really got in my face and said, 'OK, you have to calm down, you cannot let it take control. You have to breathe.' He was like an inch away from my face. But I was, 'OK sir, yes sir,' because he was an officer, so I can't punch him." In contrast, Emily, an enlisted Navy servicewoman, said that her first labor and delivery experience was "traumatic and unnecessary because of having to see a military physician." She ended up having what she viewed as an unnecessary C-section. Emily had to give birth at the Navy hospital where she worked, and, as a result, "I had to give birth in front of young men and women that I worked with on a daily basis, because I am a corpsman, and it was mortifying having them see me in such a vulnerable state." She said that for a year after the birth of her first daughter she suffered "PTSD-like symptoms (flashbacks and nightmares, anxiety attacks) when seeing this physician because I worked in the same hospital as I delivered and had anxiety attacks any time I had to walk past the labor and delivery ward." She elaborated, "Women giving birth at military hospitals are not treated well and I would never give birth at a military hospital again if I had the choice."

In the above narratives, it is clear that, although servicewomen are grateful for their low-cost health care, they also feel as if the sacrifices they make to serve in the military extend beyond the battlefield and work/life balance. Their health care is subpar, which they feel is a significant sacrifice, and they feel powerless to change it as long as they are on active duty.

RESPONSES TO THE PREGNANCY DISCOURSES:
ENACTING MACHO MATERNITY

In response to feeling patronized, punished, and powerless, servicewomen often inadvertently reinforced and sustained the dominant discourses about pregnancy in the military. Their actions illustrate Foucault's point that micropractices in society complicate hierarchical models of power relations.[20] Often negative messages about pregnancy—for example, it is inconvenient, it is a burden, it deviates from what it means to be a so-called "good" service member—are internalized by servicewomen, who then engage in self-disciplining conduct to adhere to the military's expectations. This is similar to Meisenbach and colleagues' findings that women negotiating maternity leave often internalize and then articulate discourses that limit their own agency.[21] Indeed, many interviewees suggested that they engaged these strategies to conform to notions of what it means to be an ideal servicemember. In this way, servicewomen become co-constructors of the neoliberal discourses that often serve to constrain them, rather than address and correct them, creating another circuit of discipline.

A prominent way many servicewomen attempt to mitigate the pejorative discourses surrounding pregnancy is through the liberal feminist performance of what Smithson and Stokoe call "macho maternity."[22] The term refers to taking maternity "like a man" (based on widely accepted gender scripts), or when "women feel compelled to work like men to succeed."[23] Through performances of macho maternity, women negotiate the tension between the desire for complete social equality with men and the material reality of sex differences. Smithson and Stokoe's research was based on interviews with women in banking and accounting organizations, and this term could be applied to pregnant servicewomen who continue to work as hard as they did before they were pregnant. In this sphere, servicewomen are dealing with unique tensions. Specifically, they are working hard not only because they are in the military, but, as Magellan, a senior enlisted sailor, explained, because they are *women* in the military. This is an important intersectional component of their identities, and additional facets, including rank, branch, and location also affect how servicewomen act and work during their pregnancies. Together, the following sections lend insight into the ways that the military and servicewomen cocreate a circuit of discipline that serves to reinforce the very ideologies that discriminate against servicewomen.

Working Even Harder during Pregnancy

A common phrase used by servicewomen in the interviews was that they had to "work twice as hard" as their male colleagues in order to feel equal to them—and this was *before* they were pregnant. Once servicewomen were pregnant, they often felt the need to work even harder. Part of the reason for this was because servicewomen felt an immense pressure to represent pregnant servicewomen as capable, contributing members of the military community. For example, Roxanne said, "Being in the military, I think we're always judged for being a girl. And unfortunately, I don't think that has ever changed. I feel like I've had to work at least twice as hard to get where I am than my male counterpart. So I feel like when you get pregnant, or you're having a baby, people look at you like, 'Oh, really? So now you're not going to do even more work?'" Roxanne's comments reflect the extreme pressure servicewomen feel to perform at the highest levels when they are not pregnant, and how much more pressure it brings once they are.

Magellan, a senior enlisted servicewoman, also felt equality was something she had to earn as a woman in the military, and then again as a pregnant servicewoman,

> You know in the Navy, in the military you have to do, I feel . . . I've had to do twice what the boys do so that they don't point fingers and say, "Oh, it's because you're pregnant that you don't have to do this." Or "Oh, it's because you're a girl you get away with this." Um, so, you know I feel as if I've always put forth extra effort so that I could run circles around them so that they could not say, "Oh, you know Magellan doesn't have to do this because she's, you know, whatever."

Magellan clearly explained how the military makes it difficult for women, especially pregnant women, to experience the feeling of equality due to their sex differences.

Two important factors likely influence the pressure servicewomen feel to work extra hard: the reality that women are a significant minority in the military, and that pregnant women are an even bigger minority. Alexa, an Air Force officer, recounted how she was one of two women where she was located, and the only one who was married and expecting a child, so she felt pressure to be a good example. Roxanne, a Navy pilot, explained how "I felt like I represented a big group of people, 'cause I'm the only one." Because she was the only female officer at her location, and there were only a handful of enlisted women, she explained the pressure she felt to set a good example for what a pregnant servicewoman's work ethic should entail.

Given this pressure, servicewomen often emphasized how they worked up until they delivered their babies, performing a macho maternity work ethic. For example, Magellan stated, "I worked every day and Commander Smith would come in and kick me out of the emergency room. You know, tending to patients and still trying to do everything everybody else is doing, with my cankles!" Despite her swelling ankles, Magellan continued to perform her regular duties as the equivalent of a physician's assistant. Similarly, Samantha, a junior enlisted sailor, stated, "I was working up until two days before I had my son." Joanna, a former senior enlisted Army servicewoman, noted that even when she was put on bed rest a month before each of her children was born, she would work from home via telephone. Ariel, a senior enlisted sailor, described how she went to work with contractions; she only left when her "contractions got too bad," and she delivered her baby a few hours later. Similarly, Kristen, a Navy officer, recalled working "up to the day" that she went into labor, and Navy officers Getoya and Cindy both worked until the day before they had their children (because their children were born on Saturdays). Similarly, Lynn, an Air Force officer, fought to stay in her job until her baby was born. Her squadron commander tried to move her off the flight line, and she countered by asking him to find the paperwork requiring her to do so. He could not produce the paperwork, so she stayed "until I had the baby, and I actually worked right up until the day before I had her. And I was two weeks overdue."

Roxanne said that being a pilot makes pregnancy even more difficult for one's career due to the restrictions on flying during the first and third trimesters. This is significant because it means losing flight hours toward promotion. She said that the difficulty is that the men's wives have babies, but it does not typically affect their flight hours and therefore their careers. So, to attempt to stay on an equal footing with her male peers, Roxanne fought to get a waiver to fly, since she did not qualify for her promotion before she was pregnant. As a result, with the help of a supportive skipper, she was able to obtain a waiver that allowed her to fly one hundred hours during an eighteen-day trip and qualified as an aircraft commander while pregnant.

In each of these instances, the servicewomen emphasized that they did not let their pregnancies detract from their job performances or progress toward promotions. This is especially significant, because pregnancy is a time when many women experience increased fatigue, tiredness, soreness, aches and pains, and rapid weight gain, which makes it even more difficult to ignore physical differences from men, let alone exert even more effort than before. Additionally, it was very common for officers to discuss how much more pressure they felt to continue working due to their higher rank and roles in leadership. Because there are fewer of them and they are more difficult to replace, many officers felt strong pressure to work hard and also to ignore any accommodations offered to them.

Ignoring Guidelines and Accommodations

Often pregnant servicewomen performed duties that the military advised against. For example, a few women, including Lynn, Ariel, Frida, and Magellan, were dedicated to avoiding disruptions and did not want to be treated differently, so they did not immediately report their pregnancies as early as the military guidelines require. Magellan, an enlisted Navy servicewoman working as an independent duty corpsman (the equivalent of a physician's assistant), explained that she lied to her commanding officer about how many weeks pregnant she was so that she could keep working. As she explained, "I really, really like my job, and at sixteen weeks, they take you off of the ambulances. So I fibbed and I was like, 'Oh no, I just found out I was pregnant.' I was delayed about three, maybe four, weeks." She finally fessed up to how many weeks pregnant she was after she had a very bad ambulance call, one that she should not have been on while pregnant, and it scared her to realize how she was putting herself and her unborn baby at risk.

Additionally, many servicewomen did not take advantage of accommodations offered to them. For example, Elizabeth, a Navy public affairs officer, explained that she was at a new command when she was eight months pregnant, and, despite being told she could take her time to adjust to the move, she was aware that she was making first impressions. In her words, "I worked until my water broke, and we were actually doing a command and control exercise where I was working shift work the week of my due date. There was this huge darn hill, and I had to park at the bottom of the hill and walk up the hill to the door. And on one of those walks up the hill my water broke." Elizabeth did not want the first impression her new command had of her to be that of an absentee pregnant woman, so she worked until her body went into labor to show her career dedication.

Many servicewomen also did not take advantage of accommodations in attempts to try to conform to military uniform standards, despite being given an exception due to their pregnancies. One of the recurring themes that surfaced in almost every interview was whether servicewomen were allowed to wear tennis shoes as their feet and ankles swelled due to pregnancy, making their boots uncomfortable to wear. Additionally, because boots are expensive, many women did not want to buy another size up each time their boots became too small during their pregnancies.

For Ariel, a senior enlisted servicewoman, it was important to avoid doing anything that would distinguish her as different. As she said, "I didn't play the, you know, 'I've gotta wear sneakers.' I wore my boots every day, I wore my uniform every day." For Ariel, it was important to avoid taking advantage of anything that would distinguish her as different from other sailors. Lynn, an Air Force officer, also felt this way. She said that although she could wear tennis shoes instead of combat boots, "I chose not to do that. I wore my boots." By adhering as closely as they could to the dress code, these servicewomen sought to display their equality with their male peers, exemplifying the strategy of macho maternity.

This performance of macho maternity reflects military policy discourse. For example, policies state the situations in which pregnant servicewomen in the Navy may switch to tennis shoes: "At the discretion of an HCP [health care provider], a pregnant servicewoman may be issued a tennis shoe chit, specifying the duration of wear. Tennis shoes shall be worn in an inconspicuous manner."[24] The emphasis on being "inconspicuous" reinforces the priority of the servicemembers' uniformity, despite the fact that the pregnant body alone makes women no longer uniform. Even for considerations of appropriate footwear, pregnancy is characterized as a violation of military policy despite the exceptions being made and put into policies. In response to a culture that continues to frame pregnancy this way, many servicewomen perform macho maternity in efforts to maintain equality with their male peers and avoid being labeled as less than an ideal service member. Indeed, Frida, a retired Navy officer, said that despite having the Instructions available to her, she did not pay attention to them until later in her pregnancy because, "I didn't feel like it applied to me anyway." In other words, she was not interested in the accommodations granted to her because of her pregnancy; she was going to continue to work the same way she had pre-pregnancy.

In an extreme display of macho maternity, Ariel used her physical training (PT) clothes to show her dedication, and she also continued to do PT four times each week until she delivered her son. She explained, "I mean, as far as PT clothes, you can wear your regular PT clothes and you can wear your shirt out. But I tucked it in until the day I had him and I wore my PT gear, and I could have went to civilian clothes at the end, but I didn't. Kind of a long story, 'cause I was having a hard time getting some of the other senior people from another Navy command, I couldn't get them to dress properly, so, I continued to tuck in everything and do that." Ariel gained seventy pounds while she was pregnant, and likely could not easily tuck in her shirt. Yet, her dedication to military policies meant that she adhered to them despite her discomfort, so as to set an (extreme) example for her peers.

In all of these examples, servicewomen chose not to take advantage of the policies that granted them rest or relief out of fear that it would make them stand out as different or as receiving favors. Instead, they often went to extremes enacting macho maternity to avoid such appearances.

RESISTING MACHO MATERNITY

One may argue that the performance of macho maternity is not necessarily surprising, given that those who join the military self-select, and therefore women who join the military may already be predisposed to engage in macho maternity strategies, similar to what Cindy noted in the quote opening this chapter. However, this assumption oversimplifies the issue and does not take into account the many reasons why people join the armed services, including service to country, career advancement, financial stability, health and housing benefits, college education, and more. Ultimately, macho maternity places extraordinary burdens on servicewomen that servicemen do not face. This reinforces a climate in which women's labor—both reproductive and paid—is once again undervalued compared to men's.

Similar to the previous chapter on hyperplanning, although many of the interviewees exemplified macho maternity, there were a few that showed signs of resistance. For Frida, a recently retired Navy officer, there was a tension between wanting to perform macho maternity and realizing that for the sake of her body and her baby, she needed to take a step back. As she said, especially with her fourth pregnancy, she did not want anyone to know she was pregnant until the last moment, because she did not want to be treated any differently, and she did not want anyone to think that she could not do her job well. However, when the stress of her job combined with the bodily stress and fatigue she was feeling as a pregnant servicewoman and mother of three, she said, she reached the point where she felt, "Yes, I now *do* want to be treated differently." She explained that it was difficult to manage the reality of her physical, material situation and her desire not to slow down due to the demands of her job.

Another common discussion, especially among officers, was how much they emphasized the need not to perform macho maternity when giving advice to pregnant servicewomen. For example, Alexa, an Air Force officer explained how she would tell women not to be afraid to say that they are not able to do certain duties due to their health and that of their babies. She said, somewhat self-reflectively, "I think a lot of women are hesitant because they're in such a male-dominated career field, especially with the first pregnancy, that they don't want to be seen as slackers or trying to avoid work, so that they overdo it sometimes or they don't ask for help." However, despite encouraging other women to take advantage of the policies, servicewomen often did not do it when it came to their own situations, showing how deeply ingrained macho maternity is.

CHALLENGING THE STATUS QUO

To conclude, as women continue to increase their representation as service personnel, changes are going to be necessary in terms of policies and culture. The concept of macho maternity reinforces that the increased number of women might not mean that gender equality is increasing. Rather, as Buzzanell explained over two decades ago, "increased numbers of women are insufficient for changing organizing processes because top women had to behave in promotable (masculine) ways to achieve advancement."[25] In the case of this chapter, it means women are performing macho maternity, which ultimately reinforces—rather than resists, challenges, or changes—the hypermasculine military culture. Instead of forcing women to mold to male standards, I offer some suggestions.

First, servicewomen are not one-dimensional beings; their multiple subjectivities include acting as servicemembers, mothers, friends, wives, superiors, subordinates, and the list goes on. (Of course, men, too, have multiple subjectivities, even in the "uniform" military, but that is beyond the scope of this book.) These multiple subjectivities mean that servicewomen experience contradictory ways of thinking about equality and discrimination. It is not realistic (or wise) to assume that all servicewomen think or believe the same way, even if they have experienced similar situations, like pregnancy. Instead, women should be recognized as having multiple subjectivities and be allowed the right to manage decisions regarding their bodies based on their own beliefs, circumstances, and experiences. This means commanding officers should not make career decisions for pregnant servicewomen based on their own assumptions about motherhood and pregnancy, but should consult with the pregnant servicewoman. Macho maternity also essentially ignores this reality, asking servicewomen to conform to the "uniform" and "universal" standards for "good" servicemembers—that is, male standards.

Secondly, if a majority of servicewomen, and especially those in leadership positions as officers, continue to avoid or reject the accommodations given to pregnant servicemembers, instead of reinforcing the work ethic of the pregnant women, it reinforces the idea that pregnancy is a problem. This is troublesome, because instead of welcoming women as women with their many unique biological and reproductive characteristics, it reinforces that women should only be viewed as contributing servicemembers if they are able to make their bodies perform like men's, downplaying or trying to ignore/hide those aspects that mark them as different. It also problematically contributes to the stigmatization of accommodation policies.

Additionally, the interviews indicate that there is a need for the military to once again revisit the maternity uniform. If the military really wants to make everyone appear "uniform," the maternity "tents" need to be reconsidered, as many of the servicewomen expressed that these uniforms were one of the major reasons they felt so out of place when they were pregnant. Pregnancy is stigmatized enough, and the military maternity uniform serves in some ways as a scarlet letter of sorts, a punishment for what is otherwise considered a natural part of many women's lives.

Finally, the military health care system needs to be reevaluated when it comes to prenatal care. Servicewomen are risking their lives to serve the country, and they should have access to health care that follows general health guidelines, like seeing OB doctors or midwives for their prenatal visits. Additionally, seeing the same doctor(s) for those visits will help with continuity of care. If steps are taken toward making changes like these, perhaps the belief that pregnancy and the military are incompatible—which drives performances of macho maternity—will fade.

5 Negotiating Postpartum Policies

I pumped breast milk in Iraq.

—Michelle

Miranda served fifteen years in the Navy, first as a surface warfare officer (SWO) and then as a public affairs officer. She had the first of her four children in 2007, and the end of her six-week maternity leave coincided with the start of Fleet Week. As she explained, "Fleet Week is the busiest week of the year for us. It's when the Navy pulls into New York City and all the sailors are coming off and there's all different kinds of events and activities." Stating that she "needed to be back" for Fleet Week, Miranda recalled, "So, that was a little crazy coming back to work for the first time after having a new baby." Essentially, she went from recuperating at home and breastfeeding her baby for six weeks on maternity leave to working twenty-hour days on her feet in her white dress uniform.

Babies around six weeks of age eat approximately every three hours, and nursing mothers' bodies produce milk to meet that demand. This means that every three hours or so, the mother's breasts fill with milk, and if she does not express the milk—either by breastfeeding or pumping—she will become engorged and extremely uncomfortable.

Additionally, because breast milk works via demand and supply, if the milk is not expressed at the same times that the baby would be feeding, the body stops producing as much milk. If this goes on for too long consistently, the body may stop producing milk altogether.

Feeling engorged, and aware of this breastfeeding supply reality, Miranda tried to sneak away from her post at Fleet Week to pump, but the only location she found was a "crappy dirty pier." Having no bathroom to pump, and becoming engorged standing on her feet for twelve hours, she recalls, "I felt like I was about to die. And so after Fleet Week, the nursing just stops and I had no success." Miranda's milk dried up during Fleet Week, so she was only able to breastfeed her firstborn for six weeks. In her words, her "breastfeeding success was crushed."

Miranda's story exemplifies the extreme pressures servicewomen face from two very different parts of their lives that often have competing demands. On the one hand, Miranda sees herself as a mother, and is able to—and desires to—breastfeed her baby. On the other hand, Miranda is an officer in the Navy with significant responsibilities, and she desires to fulfill her work obligations and continue to promote. The interview with Miranda, as well as with other servicewomen, quickly made it apparent that bound up within the concept of maternity leave, breastfeeding, and work, were issues of identity, most specifically around what it means to be a good military servicemember and a mother.

The military has one of the most generous maternity leave policies in U.S. society, yet, like many working mothers in the civilian sector, servicewomen continue to find these dual roles difficult to maintain as they come into tension with one another. This chapter examines this tension closer, in order to understand the factors—cultural, systemic, and personal—that contribute to it. In a culture where working moms are disciplined to be both good mothers and good workers, I find that working mothers in the U.S. military often contribute to and reinforce the very cultural norms that exacerbate the policy-culture disconnect, therefore perpetuating the circuits of discipline.

THE GOOD MOTHER VS. GOOD WORKER

Many communication scholars have researched the dialectic of the opposing good worker and good mother ideologies. On the one hand, there is the good worker identity. Acker argued that in U.S. society, the ideal worker is one who is dedicated to the job, placing it above other priorities in life, including one's personal life.[1] Additionally, Ashcraft emphasized that the ideal worker is understood to be "seemingly gender-neutral . . . a disembodied being whose sexuality, emotions, and capacity for procreation remain invisible."[2] These attributes have historically been associated with White men, and the idea that (White) men are so-called neutral and normative—and every other type of body deviates—is one of the oldest understandings about bodies.[3] This means that views of the "good worker" in both the U.S. military and the United States in general, are male- (and race-) biased, placing women always already at a disadvantage.[4]

In response to this understanding of the "universal," "good," or "ideal" worker, many women perform macho maternity, where they downplay any differences from men and attempt to "work like men" in order to be successful, as was discussed in the previous chapter.[5] As Smithson and Stokoe pointed out, because of the good worker ideology, with its implicit male bias, organizational communication scholars have noticed a "theme of women succeeding when they act 'like men.'"[6] Similarly, Blair-Loy argued that women in occupations that are traditionally male dominated (in this case, the U.S. military is a prime example), embraced a "traditionally masculine schema of devotion to work and fulfilled its strenuous demands."[7] The problem, of course, comes when these same female workers are also devoted to the schema of motherhood.

The concept of motherhood in the United Sates is laden with cultural understandings, and is studied by scholars across disciplines. Ultimately, as communication scholar Buchanan, and later O'Brien Hallstein, argued, the term *mother* and the larger concept of motherhood carry rhetorical force in that *mother* is conceived of as a "god term" in our culture that encapsulates socially acceptable ideas and ideals about women's roles, families, and our society as a whole.[8] In parsing out the concept of mothering, Adrienne Rich wrote of the distinction between the institution of motherhood and the experience of mothering. As she explained, the institution of motherhood is oppressive to women because it is defined and controlled by men. It is within the institution of motherhood that the "god term" *mother* exists and is perpetuated. In contrast, the *experience* of motherhood can be empowering for women.[9]

However, despite the god-term status of mothering and motherhood, scholars have noted that motherhood is still "low-status work" that "is part of the larger discursive formation of gender and so reiterates its governing constructs of male and female, masculinity and femininity."[10] As such, mothers are simultaneously positioned as credible authority figures and people to be admired, yet also disadvantaged by the gendered status quo.

One of the ways institutionalized motherhood is experienced today is through what Hays calls the intensive mothering ideology. Hays argues that since World War II, the "intensive mothering" ideology has emerged in which mothers are to prioritize their children above all else, spending substantial amounts of time, energy, and emotions on them.[11] An extension to intensive mothering is what Douglas and Michaels call the "new momism."[12] New momism started to gain traction in the 1980s and emphasizes that women are to be the primary caretakers of their children and are to be defined by their relationship to their children, because mothering is the ultimate job for *all* women.[13] Recently, as was mentioned in the introduction to this book, Fixmer-Oraiz theorized "homeland maternity," a pervasive ideology that emerged after 9/11 and advocates for neofifties gender roles.[14] Each of these scholars, along with Mack, argued that while these institutionalized forms of motherhood appear to celebrate mothers, they actually set up "unattainable standards of perfection that undermine women."[15]

Furthermore, scholars point out that these mothering and maternal ideologies glorify individualism and personal responsibility.[16] Although this is in line with much of the second wave of feminism's emphasis on choice, it also means that there is little or no recognition of systemic responsibility, which perpetuates unattainable intensive mothering and places sole responsibility on mothers—not society.[17] Thus, Eyer argues, "society's ills"—such as divorce rates, single motherhood, welfare, child poverty, and more—are blamed on mothers.[18] Therefore, although fathers are important when it comes to raising children, Collett argues that it is ultimately mothers who are held accountable for how the children turn out.[19] Given the nature of this ideology, which continues to dominate U.S. society, it is not surprising that O'Brien Hallstein contends that all women, whether or not they practice intensive mothering (or are even mothers), are disciplined into it.[20]

These mothering/maternal ideologies are unattainable for stay-at-home moms, and the problem is exacerbated for mothers who work. Hays refers to this as the "cultural contradictions of motherhood," or the fact that the cultural ideology of motherhood dictates that one should give oneself completely to one's child(ren), and the cultural ideology of a good worker dictates that one should give oneself completely to one's job. In reality, working mothers are trying to balance two full-time jobs.[21] O'Brien Hallstein explains this tension, stating that "intensive mothering acknowledges that gender roles and expectations have changed in the public sphere without significantly changing in terms of ongoing gender-based assumptions and expectations that mothers are still primarily responsible for childrearing and caregiving in the private sphere."[22] In order to negotiate the tension between these competing ideologies, many working mothers attempt to forge the identity of a "good working mother."[23]

Ironically, as increasingly more women have entered the workforce, the intensive mothering ideology and its associated expectations have also intensified, and along with it the myth that women are able to "have it all."[24] Yet women continue to realize that the balancing act between employment and motherhood is quite difficult, in no small part due to how U.S. society compartmentalizes private and public spheres. Historically, the private sphere has been where women and mothers belong, and men—who work—have belonged in public life. Therefore, the public/private dichotomy has always been associated with gender.[25] Yet women's presence in the workforce challenges this dichotomy. The problem, as Turner and Norwood point out, is that "The demands of the good worker are incompatible with those of good mothering, leaving working mothers to sacrifice either work for children or children for work."[26] As a result, and in attempts to manage the "cognitive acrobatics"[27] associated with the tension between the two spheres, Turner and Norwood explained how women either practice bounded or unbounded motherhood.[28] In bounded motherhood, working women suppress maternal practices that might differentiate them from their male colleagues, emulating the bodily practices of men. In unbounded motherhood, women do not try to conform to patterns of male behavior, but instead bring maternal practices (e.g., breastfeeding) into the workplace, therefore embodying the identity of "good working mothers."[29]

In all of these conversations about cultural expectations for and ideologies of good workers, good mothers, and good working mothers, the concept of identity is crucial. For many working women, and for many women in this study, there is concern that the new identity of mother will not overshadow the identity as worker. (This is noted in the previous chapter when servicewomen did not want to be viewed as "pregnant colleagues.") For example, Buchanan discovered that historically, powerful women—whether in politics, work, or elsewhere—found that their identity as mothers subsumed all other previous identities. In other words, women who become mothers are seen by others mainly as mothers, and nothing else. This is likely because of the cultural belief that a woman's ultimate role is mother.[30] Buzzanell et al. found this aspect of identity to be problematic for working mothers who have "joint allegiance" to the two historically incompatible ideologies of good worker and good mother.[31] What will become apparent in the pages that follow are the ways that identity is both self-constructed and also constructed through interactions with others.[32] Communicatively speaking, as much as women may want to control their identities, they are always already being forged in their interactions with others. Therefore, how others perceive one's identity—as a mother or a worker, in this case—can have significant impacts on how one is treated and how one views oneself.

U.S. AND U.S. MILITARY MATERNITY LEAVE POLICIES

Before moving on, it is important to contextualize the research, specifically by discussing maternity leave policies in the United States and the U.S. military. Most women in the United States—approximately 88 percent—do not receive *any* paid maternity leave.[33] In fact, a recent study found that nearly one in four employed mothers return to work within two weeks of delivering a baby because they either are not given, or cannot afford, to take time off.[34] Another study found that nearly half of mothers and fathers "didn't even take two days off work" following the birth or adoption of a child.[35] Furthermore, according to the National Compensation Survey conducted by the Bureau of Labor Statistics, only 14 percent of U.S. workers have access to any form of a paid family leave plan (which is available to both men and women and includes caring for new babies, as well as for sick family members).[36] Given these statistics, it is not surprising that the issue of paid maternity leave in the United States has been an ongoing debate in recent decades, and lately it has even seen bipartisan support.[37]

Many have criticized the United States for being the only industrialized country in the world that does not have paid family leave.[38] Within the United States, only five states have official paid leave policies, which means that workers in most of the country often rely on the Family Medical Leave Act (FMLA), which grants workers up to twelve weeks off from work, unpaid.[39] In many cases, workers use their short-term disability plans to earn 60 percent of their normal income while away from work, but for those who have worked at their current place of employment for less than one year, or for those who work at companies with fewer than fifty employees, FMLA is not even an option.[40] Additionally, when it comes to time off after having a baby, research has found that class and education make a difference in the amount of leave taken. Higher-earning women tend to work for companies that offer paid family leave plans, and women with college degrees tend to take off at least six weeks after having their babies, whereas women without college degrees often have to take significantly less.

In contrast to the general U.S. public, the U.S. military has historically offered a relatively generous paid maternity leave. Given the current state of maternity, parental, and paid family leave in the U.S. civilian sector, it comes as little surprise that most of the servicewomen interviewed—enlisted and officers alike—commented on how grateful they were for their paid maternity leave. When the initial phase of interviews took place with enlisted servicewomen in 2013, all servicewomen were granted six weeks (forty-two days) of paid maternity leave. During this leave, which was required to be taken consecutively following the birth of a child, servicewomen continued to collect their regular salary *and* accrued vacation time at the same rate as if they were working—exponentially more generous than the average U.S. organization leave program. Several of the servicewomen interviewed were thankful for this leave, especially since they were well aware that most of their civilian counterparts were lucky to be given *unpaid* time off.

On May 13, 2015, the secretary of the Navy, Ray Mabus, announced a slew of personnel changes, including initiatives regarding promotions, integrating with civilian industries, and temporary leave, as well as his desire to increase paid maternity leave from six weeks to twelve weeks.[41] In the address on talent management to midshipmen at the U.S. Naval Academy, Mabus explained that one of the primary reasons he was motivated to increase paid maternity leave was "so that people won't have to choose between family, or having a family, and service."[42] This was in line with his goal to allow for more career flexibility, which has increasingly been "seen as a key factor in future retention—especially for women—something the service must have to compete with private sector companies that can often pay more and that already provide more flexible career choices."[43]

Shortly after the address at the U.S. Naval Academy, in July 2015, Mabus announced that the Navy would be granting eighteen weeks maternity leave in an effort to better support and retain women servicemembers, as well as attract more women to serve.[44] Because women in their late twenties to mid-thirties separate from the Navy at a rate that is double that of their male peers, most often due to the desire to have more flexibility to be home with their children, this policy change was made in hopes that separations would decrease.[45] Mabus further explained that his goal with this dramatic increase was to see women comprise a quarter of every Navy fleet by the year 2025 because he believed that "a more diverse force is a stronger force."[46] He further explained, "In the Navy and the Marine Corps, we are continually looking for ways to recruit and retain the best people. We have incredibly talented women who want to serve, and they also want to be mothers and have the time to fulfill that important role the right way. We can do that for them. Meaningful maternity leave when it matters most is one of the best ways that we can support the women who serve our county. This flexibility is an investment in our people and our Services, and a safeguard against losing skilled service members."[47] Increased maternity leave may help the Navy by retaining the talents of skilled women who might otherwise leave. This is important, not only because retention stabilizes troop readiness, but also because it means that women who have already been trained and in whom the military has already invested will likely return, so that the military does not have to pay to train someone else to replace them.[48] Paid maternity leave also has physical and psychological health benefits for the mother as well as the child, as women can recover physically, emotionally, and mentally without a concern about a smaller—or no—paycheck.[49]

Indeed, Mabus's emphasis on caring first and foremost for the people in the Navy by offering flexibility was evidenced through the words of another of his statements, where he said, "When the women in our Navy and Marine Corps answer the call to serve, they are making the difficult choice to be away from their children—sometimes for prolonged periods of time—so that they can do the demanding jobs that we ask them to do.... With increased maternity leave, we can demonstrate the commitment of the Navy and Marine Corps to the women who are committed to serve."[50] With this change, the Navy became the first branch of the military to provide women with more than six weeks of paid leave by tripling it.[51] Upon closer look, Mabus's words carry extra meaning. Whereas many debates surrounding maternity matters refer to women as "mothers," Mabus continued to refer to them as "women." Through this language, Mabus was validating pregnant and parenting servicewomen's dual identities and not reducing them to a solo identity of mothers.[52] As will be discussed further in this chapter, servicewomen's identities—which include both how they see themselves and how others see them—are extremely important in discussions of maternity in the military.[53] Yet, although Mabus's discourse affirmed the dual identities of servicewomen, it simultaneously perpetuated the ideology of the good working mother, or so-called supermom, who can "have it all"—a full-time job and full-time motherhood, two identities that are much more difficult to balance in reality.[54]

The new leave policy went into effect on August 5, 2015, and applied retroactively to any woman who took maternity leave after the birth of a child since January 1, 2015.[55] In contrast to the original six week maternity leave, the additional twelve weeks did not need to be taken at once, but rather could be spread out within the first year of her child's birth.[56] Many women used this as a way to manage the transition back to work. For instance, Mae, an officer in the Navy who was given eighteen weeks, used the additional twelve-week leave to return to work slowly, by taking every Friday off over the course of one year.

According to Commander Chris Servello, a spokesperson for the chief of Naval Personnel, the change from the initially proposed twelve weeks to eighteen weeks of paid maternity leave was influenced by an announcement that Google had increased its maternity leave to eighteen weeks.[57] After this, the number of new mothers who left Google dropped by half.[58] Similar to recruiting and retention problems in the military, technology and science careers also see slightly more than 50 percent of women employees leave their fields due to issues with work-life balance. However, unlike tech companies, new moms in the military are still required to meet body fat and physical fitness standards after they give birth to a child, so the two sectors are not direct equivalencies.[59]

There were seventy-one thousand women in the Navy and Marine Corps as of January 2015, according to Defense Department data.[60] The Navy estimated that approximately five thousand women would be eligible for the "Additional Maternity Leave" (AML) benefit each year.[61] Although women are still a small percentage of the Navy, approximately 18 percent of officers and 19 percent of enlisted personnel, they now benefit from some of the most progressive policies when it comes to maternity in the United States.[62] In an interview with National Public Radio's *Morning Edition*, Jane Waldfogel, a professor at Columbia University School of Social Work, explained that while

> the military doesn't get much attention as a family-friendly employer ... they've been way ahead in terms of the quality of the child care that they offer to servicemen and women. And I think this extension of maternity leave is motivated by some of the same instincts of if you're going to recruit the best young men and women, you've got to provide them family-friendly policies. I think a few years ago people would've said, 18 weeks in the United States, you must be dreaming? And with the military doing this, this now sets a new standard which I think other companies, other employers and other employees will start paying attention to.[63]

This mutual influence of the military and civilian society, and especially, as was noted earlier, between the military and tech companies like Google, is significant. If an organization with a low percentage of female employees makes such a dramatic change, it has the potential to influence other organizations and create larger cultural change for U.S. workers.

However, the generous eighteen-week leave did not last long. By February 2016, the Navy had to roll back its maternity leave to twelve weeks, after Secretary of Defense Ash Carter (who outranks Ray Mabus as secretary of the Navy), announced that all branches would get twelve weeks of paid maternity leave, because he "thought it was important that we have the same standard across the joint force."[64] He added that, "Twelve weeks is extremely generous and puts us in the top tier of American employers," and explained that the reason he did not change it to eighteen weeks is because "you have to balance that against the readiness costs associated with it."[65] In other words, to Carter, the military can afford to have women absent for twelve weeks, but at eighteen weeks, military operations and national security would start to suffer.

The military-wide twelve-week maternity leave policy was announced with what Carter called his "Force of the Future" initiative—which was very similar to Mabus's previously mentioned Talent Management address approximately four months earlier—that listed changes the secretary of defense hoped would help better the lives of (and therefore retain) servicemembers and also be attractive to potential candidates for the U.S. military.[66] Other family-related announcements made by Carter included a pilot program that would pay for the freezing of active-duty servicemembers' eggs and sperm (but would not pay the full cost of IVF).[67] Carter further explained that these changes are necessary because "women at peak ages for starting a family leave the military at the highest rates."[68] The hope was that when servicewomen had the opportunity to freeze eggs with no out-of-pocket cost, they would be willing to delay pregnancy.

What goes unsaid and is largely ignored or overlooked in these changes and announcements is a recognition of unplanned pregnancies. As was discussed in previous chapters, even with the best planning and use of birth control methods, pregnancies can happen, and medical failures do occur.[69] Therefore, while the option to freeze eggs might appeal to some, it does not solve issues related to unplanned pregnancies. Additionally, asking women to freeze their eggs, and ultimately have children at an older, so-called "high-risk advanced maternal age," includes other compromises and complications.[70] And, of course, there is always the underlying issue that men in the military are not asked to delay childbirth or family planning, but women are.

Although the Navy was to reduce its maternity leave from eighteen to twelve weeks, all women who were pregnant or delivered by March 3, 2016, would be given the eighteen-week leave.[71] The changes in the Navy's policies are especially significant for this research project. Because of the timing of the second round of interviews for this study, and due to the nature of snowball sampling methods, a majority (fifteen out of eighteen) of the officers interviewed were in the Navy, and four of them—Getoya, Elsa, Mae, and Roxanne—fell into the group of servicewomen who were pregnant and/or had babies during the window of time where Navy servicewomen were given eighteen weeks maternity leave.

To be sure, many women in the military applauded both policy changes; however, there was skepticism from many women that taking such a significant amount of time away from their jobs would not ultimately hurt their careers; they would surely miss assignment and promotion chances while on leave. Under the military's Defense Officer Personnel Management Act (DOPMA), the branches were mandated to adopt an "up or out" policy, in which servicemembers must meet certain requirements in a specific amount of time in order to be promoted and remain in the military.[72] DOPMA made career paths predictable. However, similar to many women in academia who have children before tenure and worry about their ticking tenure clock, taking time away from servicewomen's careers for the birth of a baby could mean the end of their careers, too.[73] To assuage these fears, Carter assured, "No member shall be disadvantaged in her career, including limitations in her assignments (except in the case where she voluntarily agrees to accept an assignment limitation), performance appraisals, or selection for professional military education or training, solely because she has taken maternity leave."[74]

It is with this backdrop of changes in maternity policies that I now turn to servicewomen's postpartum experiences. I did not include questions about servicewomen's postpartum experiences in my interview protocol. However, because maternity experience is a continuum, postpartum themes were recurrent. Specifically, in this chapter I address the themes of maternity leave, breastfeeding, childcare, and physical readiness tests.[75] In each of these areas, we can see how the working mothers attempted to "have it all" and often experienced the cultural contradictions of motherhood.

MACHO MATERNITY LEAVE

The macho maternity performances discussed in chapter 4 continued during postpartum experiences, in the form of what I call "macho maternity leave," where servicewomen essentially took maternity leave "like a man." Macho maternity leave is rooted in the masculine and patriarchal American ideology of the industrious warrior. Writer Joanna Weiss focused on this ideology when she wrote about why CNN journalist Chris Cuomo, who was suffering from COVID-19 symptoms at home in early 2020 (including, but not limited to, hallucinations, restless sleep, and rapid weight loss), continued to broadcast live from his basement despite doctors recommending he rest.[76] We also see it at work in professional athletes who continue to compete while seriously injured. This type of devotion to one's job and workplace, often at great personal sacrifice, is highly praised in U.S. society as an exemplary work ethic.

Unsurprisingly, this ideology also permeates the U.S. military, and it is why it was extremely important to the servicewomen interviewed that they maintain their identities as good workers after they gave birth (mirroring the example of Yahoo executive Marissa Mayer, discussed in the first chapter, who was back in the office two weeks postpartum). It might be argued that women do not want to be seen as "good working mothers" at work, but rather only as good workers, separating the two parts of their lives. An ideology of the intensive (industrious warrior) worker seemed to influence postpartum behaviors of interview participants, such as taking shortened maternity leaves and waiving deferred deployment after giving birth. In these ways, we can see the perpetuation of servicewomen's roles as cocreators in the circuit of discipline, as they did not utilize many of the postpartum benefits available to them. In fact, in their efforts to "have it all," servicewomen often undermine the very policies put in place to accommodate them, which can also have a negative effect of further framing those who do use the benefits as weak or escaping obligations.[77] Furthermore, the concept of "macho maternity leave" wherein women "take maternity leave like a man" is inherently contradictory, essentially functioning to erase the biological, physical, and emotional changes women experience during labor and delivery and postpartum, which are the only reasons the maternity policies exist in the first place.

One way that servicewomen took maternity leave like a man was via promoting while they were on maternity leave. Elizabeth, a Navy officer, was promoted to O-5 while she was on maternity leave with her second baby, and she said that she "came in off maternity leave just to do the promotion ceremony and then went home." Similarly, Paige, a Navy officer, was on maternity leave when she received her O-4 promotion. She said that to her, the most amazing part was that she fit into her uniform for the ceremony. Frida, an officer in the Navy, was actually in the hospital with her newborn twins when her admiral called and said, "Congratulations with the twins. Boy, this is your day, Lieutenant Commander." She said that receiving the call in the hospital from her admiral who addressed her by her new rank on the day she had her twins was great. For all three women, the ability to be recognized for their achievements while on maternity leave was gratifying and affirmed that their pregnancies had not compromised their identities as good workers.

In other cases, macho maternity leave was evident by how much maternity leave servicewomen took. Despite a policy that mandated paid maternity leave, many of the servicewomen did not take all of the time given, whether it was six, twelve, or eighteen weeks. It is here where differences in rank, and specifically between enlisted servicewomen and officers, made a difference. Claudia explained how the level of responsibility she had in her position as an officer in the Navy kept her from taking a real maternity leave when she had her second child. She discussed how she was one of two people running her department, and the other person had to leave for an augmentation in Afghanistan. As a result, she was in charge of the department, and she "took the six weeks and I worked from home. I had a laptop and I was working from home the entire time even though I was technically on medical leave. Then I came back immediately after." Miranda, a Navy officer, took fewer weeks leave than she was allotted, as well, because she felt she needed to be back during Fleet Week, as was explained in the opening of this chapter. Elsa was similar with her maternity leave, taking only six weeks off instead of the allowed eighteen. She even told her colleagues to call or text her if needed while she was gone. She explained that, although this was "probably mostly self-pressure . . . it just felt like the right thing to do." Elsa said that going back after six weeks was very tough, because just getting out of the house on time with an infant is stressful. But she said that she put a lot of pressure on herself because

> I didn't want people to think, "Oh, she had a baby and now she's just kind of not as great an officer and she's not living up to the standards that she used to," so I wanted to kind of make it look like nothing had

happened. . . . I think females in general probably put more pressure on themselves than anyone else; but especially in the military, you have mostly men around you and you never want to single yourself out as a woman in a negative way. I believe that you kind of have to live to a higher standard; there have been a lot of accommodations, a lot of changes in the military, but you still kind of have to live to a higher standard, more professionalism, more just proving yourself constantly, so that's just one more way that you kind of need to show, "I still have it."

Although both Claudia and Elsa went back to work prematurely, Elsa's struggle to maintain her good worker identity is evident in her words. To her, it was important that her colleagues thought she was the "same person," not someone who had changed due to pregnancy and motherhood.[78] Buzzanell et al. found that identity struggles for managerial and professional women are "particularly acute" because of the need to juggle a "joint allegiance to traditionally incompatible ideologies (motherhood and career)."[79] Elsa's case is a prime example of this.

Kristen, a Navy officer, voiced similar feelings. She brought her newborn to work so that she could brief her boss for the president's upcoming visit. She said she brought her baby carrier around to meetings and set it next to her while she answered emails, "because it was my responsibility [to get work done]." Michelle, a Navy officer, also remembers bringing her sick child to work, because she did not feel like she could take the day off. When her child threw up, she was asked to go home. These stories are filled with the rhetoric of neoliberalism and responsibilization as the servicewomen felt ultimate responsibility themselves to manage work and childcare obligations. Douglas and Michaels explained that this societal pressure ultimately communicates, "The buck stops with you, period, and you'd better be a superstar."[80] The community/individual tension surfaces here, as servicewomen feel solely responsible for letting down their team or community. In these narratives, it becomes clear that although Mabus talked about putting flexible mechanisms in place that granted servicewomen time away from work, the cultural ideologies that the servicewomen have adopted influence their behavior and hesitancy and unwillingness to accept and take maternity leave. This can be seen in how Elsa equates being a woman as always already being a negative attribute in the military, noting how she did not want to stand out as a woman "in a negative way," which implies that a positive way to be a woman is to make sure gender and biology are not apparent. Thus, many servicewomen ignore the policies—for which many women in the United States are fighting in their own organizations—and reinforce and perpetuate a culture that devalues maternity, cocreating the circuit of discipline.

Yet, although Elsa argued her work ethic was mainly self-imposed, others explained the stigma associated with maternity leave was also influential. Emily, an enlisted servicewoman, said that many of the men thought that the six weeks women received for maternity leave was "excessive" because the woman could "sit around and do nothing all day." She said, in reality, she had C-sections with both of her babies and needed the time for her body to heal and recover. Lynn, an Air Force officer, remembers returning to work and being told, "Oh my gosh, you were gone for so long." She was also asked, "How did you enjoy your break?" She said that she was most offended by that comment, responding, "I didn't sleep, I was healing half the time." Although she did not take the full twelve weeks she was given, she said that people would have had to accept it, because it is policy. Yet, she countered that just because it's policy, "it's still looked down upon.... And then there's always going to be that question—granted, nobody asked me—but I've heard that question before of, 'Well, when women get pregnant, they get three months off automatically, so how many women get pregnant on purpose?'" This question is one that comes up often and infuriates many servicewomen for two primary reasons.[81] First, the time off after having a baby is not a vacation, but a time filled with pain, healing, and lack of sleep as they adjust to life with a newborn. Second, having a baby is not about getting three months off, but accepting a lifetime of commitment to raising a child.

Furthermore, many of the participants described how they actually received more judgment from women than they did from men. For example, Getoya, a Navy officer, explained how she was one of the few who received eighteen weeks maternity leave, and she took it. She recalls being told by other women, "You don't need it. It's selfish to take it. I can't believe that you're staying on leave with your child." Elizabeth, a retired Navy public affairs officer, attributed this to the "pride of suffering trope," explaining that older women may not have received any paid maternity leave, or perhaps just a little, and therefore believed that current women do not need it and should not receive it either. As Anne-Marie Slaughter explained it, "It's human nature to absorb the values and practices of the system that we survived and succeeded in and to demand that others make it the same way."[82] Therefore, because older servicewomen had been fine with the little leave they took, they believed women today would be fine, too. However, just because women made it work does not mean that it was right or good.

Finally, macho maternity leave also manifested when women waived their right to deferred deployment in order to progress in their careers. Although the Navy policy is that servicewomen cannot deploy or go on training within the first year of the birth of their child, servicewomen can waive their right to this policy. Frida, a Navy officer, did this, when she chose to deploy shortly after her baby was born because it felt like the best option available to her. If she had waited to deploy until her baby was one year old, she would have been gone twelve months in a war zone. Instead, she was sent to a noncombat area. Similarly, Claudia, who enlisted and then became an officer, traveled for a month of training (Training Duty or TDY that takes servicemembers away from home for extended amounts of time) while her baby was still breastfeeding. Because there are certain TDYs that must be met in order for a career to stay on track, Claudia waived the TDY portion and was grateful that no one tried to talk her out of it. In contrast, Lynn was on TDY when her daughter was four months old, and, although she tried to fight it, it still happened.

In all of these examples of macho maternity leave, individual responsibility is emphasized, reinforcing the cultural belief that managing careers and childcare are the sole responsibility of women.[83] As these women work to exhibit behaviors of unencumbered servicemembers, they simultaneously perpetuate problematic cultural beliefs, namely not taking advantage of leave that they are granted. This reflects what Meisenbach et al. found in their research: that women often internalize and then articulate maternity leave discourses that limit their own agency.[84] Indeed, many of the servicewomen in my research who attempted to conform to notions of what it means to be an ideal servicemember while on maternity leave in many ways became co-constructors of the neoliberal discourses that often serve to constrain them. When this happens, change in culture and policies is much more difficult, and when servicewomen do decide to take the leave and accommodations afforded them, they are scrutinized.

BREAST IS BEST

In addition to macho maternity leave, many of the interviews focused on breastfeeding and pumping. While most servicewomen worked intensely to maintain their "good worker" identities, several simultaneously made efforts to create and reinforce their good mother identities by finding time to breastfeed or pump when returning to work. Because of the public emphasis on "breast is best" and campaigns that encourage mothers to breastfeed their babies due to the nutritional value associated with it, breastfeeding is a key component of intensive mothering identity.[85] Although given much public attention and support, it should be noted that in the "feminist discursive space" there are disagreements over the support of "breast is best."[86] A leading feminist voice criticizing the promotion of breastfeeding is Joan B. Wolf, who questions the science behind the claims.[87] Other feminists, like Koerber (and the lactation experts she cites) support it. Despite disagreements about the science promoting "breast is best," both sides acknowledge that, for the most part, the medical community and general U.S. culture instruct women to breastfeed. Yet, as Koerber points out, there is often a disconnect between the instructions to breastfeed and the lack of accommodations to facilitate breastfeeding/pumping in the workplace.

Fortunately, for servicewomen returning from maternity leave who desire to continue breastfeeding, the military has policies in place that dictate accommodations for nursing mothers. These policies distinguish the military from other institutions, since lactation rooms at places of employment are rare in the civilian sector.[88] They are also important because they helped many women interviewed for this research negotiate the tension between needing to be at work and wanting to continue breastfeeding their babies.

Specifically, the policies as listed in OPNAV 6001.C, the Navy's Instruction that was in place at the time of the interviews, spoke favorably of making accommodations for breastfeeding.[89] Using language that emphasized medical and scientific research, Section 209(a)(1–2) states,

> (1) Breastfeeding offers proven health benefits for infants and mothers. Providing accommodations for breastfeeding offers tremendous rewards for the DOD and the Navy, in cost savings for health care, reduced absenteeism, improved morale and servicemember retention. Challenges in the workplace include lack of break time and inadequate facilities for pumping and storing breast milk. Many of these workplace challenges can be reduced with a small investment of time and flexibility.
>
> (2) DOD has directed that active and selected reserve component members be physically and mentally fit to carry out their missions and that the emphasis will be placed on the achievement of the Department of Health and Human Services' Healthy People Goals. . . . Support of servicewomen who continue breastfeeding their infant(s) upon return to duty aligns with DOD policy, ensures the physical and emotional well-being of servicewomen and their families, reduces absence from work due to illness, and improves operational readiness.[90]

At face value, this policy is very generous, recognizing the need for flexibility, and the ways that accommodating nursing mothers who return to work can ultimately help servicewomen, and the organization as a whole. The policy cites immunological benefits of breastfeeding, such as the health of the baby, as a justification for providing accommodations, because if the babies are healthier, their mothers will have to take less time off of work. It also references the positive effects of accommodations on women's physical and mental health.

Similar to the language and tone of the Navy policies, several servicewomen explained that they breastfed their babies because they knew that it was the "right" thing to do given the research and the guidelines on breastfeeding. For example, Mae, a Navy officer, believed that breastfeeding was best, for health and financial reasons. She said that she thought that the Navy was also coming to see the benefits, too: "military medical as a whole is recognizing that the health benefits of breastfeeding are gonna save money in the long run—they provide the facilities and the support so women can breastfeed; it's gonna save them money in the long run because the babies will be healthier." Likewise, toward the end of the interview, Clementine, an Air Force officer, brought up breastfeeding, stating it was "definitely very important to me . . . [because] the research is out there in truckloads as far as how beneficial it is, so I definitely wanted to, I was committed to it." Cindy, a retired Navy officer, explained that while she enjoyed breastfeeding her child, she "hated pumping," but she did it anyway because "I knew it was the right thing to do. My mom did it for me. . . . Of course I'm going to do it. It's the right thing to do for the baby. It's the right thing—it's definitely terrific. Have to do it." To Cindy, there wasn't a choice, and she was willing to be uncomfortable if she was doing something that would benefit her baby. Cindy's decision to pump despite hating it exemplifies how maternity culture often glorifies pain as "dutiful and necessary."[91]

In addition to supporting the medical community's general promotion of breastfeeding, the Navy also gave specific recommendations for how long to breastfeed. OPNAV 6001.C Section 209(a)(2) continues, "Per current professional standards, the military medical community advises pregnant servicewomen to exclusively breastfeed for the first 6 months and encourages them to continue to provide breast milk for the remainder of the first year."[92] Using the strong language of "advises," the Navy policy cites scientifically proven benefits of breastfeeding and officially recommends that working nursing mothers breastfeed for six to twelve months. Therefore, section 209(b) that follows lists how the military will accommodate that recommendation, explaining that servicewomen should be given the time (but kept to a "minimum . . . amount of time required for milk expression") and space needed to pump, which includes a place with access to water and is "a clean, secluded space (not a toilet space)."

Many servicewomen interviewed were aware of the recommendations for breastfeeding, and the most extreme case of following the guidelines for how long to breastfeed was Michelle, a retired Navy officer, who breastfed and pumped for twenty months with her first child and twenty-two months with her second. As she explained, "I'm like, the World Health Organization says two years; I'm going for two years, baby." In a memorable statement cited at the opening of this chapter, Michelle said, "I pumped breast milk in Iraq." Breastfeeding for nearly two years with each child meant that she found herself traveling for work to places like Iraq and across the United States while still pumping. Sometimes she would pump, freeze the milk, and bring it back in a suitcase, and other times she would use her own money to ship it back home on dry ice. In Iraq, she did not ship the milk home, but would pump every three hours to maintain her milk supply, and then, "walking to the porta-potty and throwing [the milk] down because there was no sink in the place I was staying."

Miranda, a Navy officer, also said that she shipped her breast milk back home when she was traveling. Similar to how Michelle would bring her milk home in a suitcase, Miranda recalled, "I was nursing when I was away from them twice and I pumped and brought back a suitcase full of milk on the plane. Oh, I also know how to ship breast milk through FedEx, too, with dry ice, it's a crazy procedure."

She explained that if women decide they want to breastfeed their babies, "it's totally doable, you just have to make sure that it works for you and for your family." Despite the ability to ship breast milk and pump in other locations, Michelle said it was frustrating to try and balance pumping with her job. She remembered driving from Virginia Beach to Washington, D.C., with her boss who was a SEAL commander, as well as a few others who were going to brief the Office of Naval Intelligence. She said that it was a three-hour drive, and she had to ask to stop for a pumping break on the way. Another time in Iraq, her group was waiting for a helicopter to take them to another location, and because she was pumping, she was burning more calories and was therefore very hungry, so she ran to the store quickly to get some food. When she returned, she was late "and the pilot of the helicopter chewed me out and I just [fake yells] 'I'm a fucking nursing mother.' [laughter] I'm like, this is not the time and the place; he doesn't want to hear that. So, instead, I said, 'Yes, my bad, I wasn't here.' So, I'm like, I got it, I'm just going to take it, I don't think it's right but this is not the time to go forth on why you are not understanding the big picture. Because yeah, it was a war zone and okay." Michelle's account echoes Elsa's words earlier about not wanting to draw attention to any of her distinctly female activities, which can be viewed as negative, despite the emphasis on the positive attributes of breast milk noted in the Navy's policies.

As some of these stories show, just because breastfeeding is viewed as good, it does not mean it is convenient or easy. It became apparent that despite military policies in place, adherence to the policies depended on many variables, including the branch of the military, rank, location, and type of job. What Michelle and Miranda do not mention is that, as officers, they had more means to ship their milk on dry ice out-of-pocket compared to enlisted servicewomen, who may not have the financial ability to do so. In each of these examples, the dedication to their role as mothers is equally as intense as their dedication to their identities of good workers.

Many women found it fairly easy to make the transition back to work, use the accommodations granted to them as nursing mothers, and therefore fulfill their work and maternal duties. Joanna, a retired enlisted Army servicewoman, had a good balance between work and pumping/breastfeeding. Shortly after she had her son, she was assigned the job of a recruiter at a Reserve center, which allowed her consistent and predictable work hours. She was able to pump at work as well as visit the day care next door to nurse her son on her lunch breaks, if she wanted to do so. Similarly, Clementine was grateful to have the support of her leadership. They did not pressure her to get back in the cockpit and fly the helicopter for the six months she was back to work before going on Career Intermission Program (CIP). She said that allowed her to continue to breastfeed and pump, which she would not have been able to do otherwise. She detailed how each flight requires body armor that is a heavy plate on the chest, and the flight is a minimum of three hours in the air and some time afterward, which would end up being a six-hour window with no chance to pump. Given the time frame for breastfeeding I discussed in the beginning of this chapter, it is easy to see how this could be problematic. Similarly, Mae expressed how grateful she was to work for the military while she was pregnant and postpartum. She said that because of all the policies, which cannot be violated, "I can't have worked in an organization that would have been a better situation to be pregnant and for post-birth." Although Mae's words are technically correct—the policies cannot be violated by the military—it has already been noted how this does not always happen in terms of how often servicewomen themselves violate the policies.

Others, primarily officers, however, found the ability to follow breastfeeding guidelines and pump at work more difficult. Claudia explained that as an officer, "you get more responsibility. It's harder to take time out of your day. It's harder to miss meetings. So people are less sympathetic for you doing that." Claudia's words reflect how "a breastfeeding worker occupies a particularly liminal space between" the good mother and the good worker ideologies because, as Payne and Nicholls point out, "workers who breastfeed have the potential to deviate from [work] norms and disrupt the 'good worker' construct simply by attending to the nutritional needs of their infants in their workplace and work time."[93] Indeed, often the demands of the job, despite a policy that said they'd be given time for milk expression, caused servicewomen to skip pumping sessions, and, because of the demand-and-supply nature of breast milk, many servicewomen's bodies stopped producing milk. Furthermore, this pressure is in direct violation of OPNAV 6001.C 201(5), which says, "The policies will ensure that the work environment supports and respects servicemembers who engage in healthy behaviors such as breast milk expression. The policies will prohibit harassment and discrimination of breastfeeding servicewomen."[94]

As an example, Frida explained how she used to be very dedicated to pumping. She pumped for nine months with her twins, and then she said the time decreased with her subsequent two children. The reason for the changes, she explained, was the different locations and jobs she had when her children were born. When she was working in New York, she had her own office, so she was able to pump while continuing to do the tasks of her job. As she explained,

> You talk about your multitasking, but I had figured out how to with those nursing bras, like stick the cones on and have—you'd hold it there long enough for suction and then I'd button my shirt up. And so, I wasn't just sitting out like this. And then I'd stick the pump itself [makes whomp noises] in the desk drawer and I mean I would type. I would type. I'd be on the phone because—and again, I had my own office so I could do this and it was great, and I got those little wipey wipes so I mean I didn't have to run to the bathroom all the time [to clean the supplies].

Frida's recollection of her pumping experience in New York explains many of the reasons pumping at work can be difficult. It requires time away from the desk if there is no option to shut the door, the pump can make loud noises, which can be distracting to colleagues and draw unwanted attention to servicewomen, and after pumping, the time to clean the pump supplies adds additional time away from work.

All of these reasons made it difficult for her to pump at her job in Washington, D.C. She explained that because she was working ten- to twelve-hour days, and needing to pump four times a day, it was taking her away from work too much (as she said, "Away from the desk physically for almost forty minutes. Times four times a day?"). So, she would sometimes skip a pumping session, and, as she said, "As soon as you skip one, it doesn't—there's no backsies. It just starts—your body goes, 'Oh, you don't need it.' And I want to say, 'No I do need it, I just didn't have the time." As a result, she lost her milk earlier than she had wanted with her subsequent two children.

Frida was not the only one whose milk dried up due to work duties. Lynn had planned to breastfeed her daughter until she was six months old, but a stressful week at work when her daughter was four months old caused her milk to dry up. She had tried to pump three times a day while she was at work, but "it seemed like every day something different was coming up," so pretty soon she was only pumping twice a day, and then there was a week where she could not find time to pump at all. She started to panic, afraid she would lose her milk. She ran out of extra pumped milk at home, and ran out of milk to send to the daycare. Out of desperation, she went home and pumped throughout the night, trying to get her supply back. She fed her daughter formula at home and sent what little she pumped overnight to day care. The next week, her milk dried up. In another example, Paige was pumping at work, but then was sent off to the Navy Academy for a short assignment. When she arrived, they only had a woman's restroom, and no designated place to pump, so she gave up breastfeeding. Claudia recalled how she "ended up drying up much earlier than I wanted to" with her first child because there was no pumping space provided. As a result, she said that she ended up in a bathroom stall with a battery pack to fuel her pump instead of an outlet. The battery pack did not supply enough power to pump effectively, so her milk dried up.

When job duties make it difficult to continue to breastfeed, we see how "organizational norms and values exact control over women's bodies and identities."[95] In this case, the demands of the military schedule meant that breastfeeding was not the main priority. Despite policies that advocated breast milk expression as healthy and encouraged it up to one year, the culture and climate of the U.S. military didn't support the policies, and a disconnect meant that the servicewomen often ended up choosing work over pumping, even though the policies granted them time and access.

This lack of balance between work and pumping happened often. For Claudia's second pregnancy, the pressures of her job "drove me to stop breastfeeding early." Specifically, when one of her coworkers started a department meeting in her absence because she was pumping, she realized that, to her, it was more important not to miss meetings than to not miss a pumping session. This competitive attitude was especially emphasized by Lynn and Getoya, both surface warfare officers (SWOs). Lynn said, "we tend to eat our own," and Getoya stated, "they say SWOs eat their young." What both women meant by this was that in their line of work, they often experienced even less support from fellow females when they were pregnant and nursing, because often the women would think, "Oh good, she's going to get pulled out of her job, so that's more options for me" (Lynn).

Each of these stories shows how the pressures of the job often conflicted with the cultural pressures of intensive mothering—in this case providing babies with breast milk. Women's bodies were required in two places at once—in their offices with colleagues and in the pump rooms. This is also an example of the public and private spheres colliding. Whereas Paige was not shy about her need to pump, putting a sign on the storage closet door where she pumped that said, "Pumping in progress," others, like Lynn, wanted to keep the two spheres separate. Turner and Norwood explained how difficult the separation of work and motherhood is with "maternal, lactating bodies" because "maternal and professional embodiment" are not able to be compartmentalized like they may be at other times in a woman's life.[96] As

Lynn tried to keep these spheres separate, she described how she had "really stressful days" and "hard hours, and pumping is not easy." She said there were countless times when someone would knock on her door while she was pumping, and she would shout, "Just a minute!" because she was too embarrassed to say she was pumping. She said that even though it was not something to be embarrassed about, she "kind of was." She was so concerned that she would skip pumping in order to attend meetings with the commander because she did not want to be "that woman" who would have to say she could not make a meeting because she needed to pump. She was very mindful so that people would not need to pick up her slack. Although Lynn may have been trying to keep up the good worker identity, Payne and Nicholls warned that this type of behavior serves to further marginalize breastfeeding in the workplace.[97]

Koerber discussed how sociocultural dynamics can often actively discourage or sabotage efforts to breastfeed and pump, even when policy states otherwise.[98] She argued that the scientific rhetoric that used a vocabulary of immunology to support breast milk as uniquely beneficial to infants' and babies' health works to degender breast milk and thus separate it from reality and the actual practice that includes women's lactating bodies. This disconnect, then, is reflected in cultures, such as the U.S. military's, where the benefits of breast milk are advocated in policy, but actual time off work or away from work to express said milk for the babies is not as supported as it should be.

The stigma many women felt when they said they needed time and space to pump was frustrating, because pumping is not a break, it's another type of (unpaid) labor. Michelle was especially frustrated with the stigma, given that, "The military supports people smoking and going to the smoke room every hour; if we can let guys go smoke, which is not good for them, we can let women do this." Paige echoed this sentiment, explaining that she and some of the nursing women would say they were going for a smoke break when they were leaving to pump so that people would not be awkward and uncomfortable or question them. She said that it was ironic, because pumping is "even less socially acceptable than smoking."

For those like Michelle, who were able to pump at work, finding satisfactory spaces to pump sometimes proved to be an issue. First of all, although there are policies about providing pumping rooms, most people in the military are unfamiliar with what the documents say and/or do not read them until they are pregnant. Therefore, many of the servicewomen found themselves in commands that did not know that pump rooms were required. Michelle recalled the policy that came out in 2008 for the Navy mandating that "each command will provide a lactation room where you can go pump, and it's not supposed to be the bathroom." She said for both pregnancies she had to show the policies to her bosses, and they said, "We had no idea that existed." They were supportive and made the needed changes. Clarissa, an enlisted Air Force servicewoman, explained that the Air Force must provide time and space during the day to visit the baby and breastfeed or to pump, and that servicewomen are "not expected to do it in a restroom." Despite these policies that mandated designated rooms for pumping, there were three main places that servicewomen mentioned pumping: in bathrooms (Claudia, Sadie, Paige, Clementine), in closets (Cindy, Elsa, Getoya), and in designated rooms (Elizabeth, Mae, Frida, Paige, Michelle). In fact, Claudia explained how, although "there is an Instruction that said that you have to provide room to pump, there wasn't [a room provided]."

Many of those who did not pump in designated rooms did not necessarily find it to be problematic. For example, both Cindy and Elsa pumped in closets and were fine with it. Cindy said that she had to walk through one man's personal workspace to get to the closet, but that it was not a problem. Although she was a little self-conscious about it, she said, "you gotta do what you gotta do." Elsa said that her closet "wasn't anything luxurious but it was fine, it was adequate, it was healthy and it was sanitary and everything."

Michelle, a Navy officer, and Clementine, an Air Force officer, pumped in bathrooms. Even though they both had to pump in bathrooms, they still kept others in mind, and how they would be affected. For example, Michelle remembers going on business trips and having to pump while sitting on a chair in the bathroom because, "I don't want to tie up one of the two stalls for forty minutes." This meant she did not have privacy while pumping, and said that she felt like saying to the women who walked in to use the restroom, with her sitting and pumping by the door, "Just pay no attention to me, ladies. Nothing to see here." Clementine did not push back about the lack of a designated pumping space because she felt that she needed to "pick her battles." She explained that because she works in a male-dominated field (she is a helicopter pilot for the Air Force, which is more male-dominated than most of the military), and because she was the only person that would need a pump room, she felt bad displacing someone from their office so she could pump every few hours. As she said, "Everybody's going to know what I'm doing, when I'm doing it, and I'm inconveniencing all these people." She further elaborated that, because there were so few females where she was located, and in her field in general, the bathrooms were "actually really clean. They would clean them with chlorine and bleach and stuff, and because there are so few females in my squadron, that honestly ended up being the most quiet and relaxing place to go."

Just as Michelle and Clementine did not want to inconvenience others, Lynn discussed how she found it a bit difficult to fight for a pumping room when only fifteen of the two hundred people working there were females, and most of them were not pregnant. Military policies require pumping spaces to be provided at locations with more than fifty employees. However, when the ratio of women to men is so low, providing a room for one woman made some servicewomen feel like it was asking too much and taking away space that could be used in a way that benefits more servicemembers.

In contrast to these situations where there were no designated rooms, was the Pentagon, a location that Elizabeth, Frida, Mae, and Paige emphasized was a wonderful place to be a nursing mother. Elizabeth described it: "The Pentagon is just the most amazing place to be pregnant and have a baby. They have the nursing mothers' rooms in every corridor of the Pentagon, where they have hospital-grade pumps, and you can post the pictures [of your babies]." Paige agreed with this, explaining that the rooms "made it really easy and it just made such a difference in being able to keep nursing." In addition to having hospital-grade pumps and refrigerators, the rooms also offered comradery for the servicewomen. Elizabeth explained how many women would get to know each other because they were on the same pumping schedule. Frida agreed that the pumping rooms offered a place to build relationships, explaining that officers and enlisted servicewomen would talk, share pictures, and share experiences and advice. In many ways, Mae explained how pumping became an equalizer, where different branches, officers, enlisted servicewomen, and civilians would get to know each other.

All of these stories show how the ability to "have it all"—being a good mother and a good worker—depend greatly on the branch, job, location, command, and colleagues one has in the U.S. military. While some were able to breastfeed for up to two years, or were able to experience comradery with other nursing mothers at the Pentagon, others found their milk drying up due to the competing demands of their jobs and their breastfeeding schedules. When women would not advocate for themselves, and/or were in a location where the command was unfamiliar with the policies, servicewomen struggled to balance pumping and working. Additionally, even if the command was on board, the culture among colleagues could sabotage efforts to continue to pump.

CHILDCARE STRUGGLES

Childcare was also a struggle for many servicewomen when they returned to work from maternity leave. The issues related to childcare are not unique to servicewomen, since approximately half of all U.S. families report difficulties in finding childcare.[99] Dual career families compose approximately 66 percent of the population and are in need of childcare, yet many times issues related to cost, availability, and quality of childcare arise.[100] In many cases across the United States, this means that parents, and often the mothers, have to make sacrifices, whether it is quitting a job, not taking a job, or changing a career trajectory in order to find a situation where childcare works.[101]

In response to childcare issues affecting their work, a group of working mothers at Amazon, the self-titled Momazonians who are approximately two thousand in number, confronted CEO Jeff Bezos in March 2019 asking for help with childcare.[102] Specifically, they were asking for policies similar to other tech giants like Apple and Google who subsidize backup childcare when the primary care arrangements fall through. Often, when there are childcare issues, mothers are the ones who shoulder the burden and make sacrifices, which may be why it has been reported that U.S. women are not entering the workforce in the numbers that were seen in the 1990s.[103]

As it was stated earlier, the military is often put in the same category as tech companies when it comes to women and careers. Both are historically male-dominated institutions, and both have recently been looking for ways to recruit and retain women. A significant difference, of course, is that the military life seeps into other areas of one's life, like physical fitness, which will be discussed shortly. There is also the reality of dual military families, where both parents are in the military and could be deployed, often leaving one parent at home to coordinate childcare and career. Candee explained that her "anxiety returning to work . . . was further complicated by the fact that I was married to an active-duty member, and his deployments, and figuring out when—'I just had the baby. I'm returning to work. When is he leaving?'" Despite some of these challenges, for many interviewed, including Tanya, Elsa, Master Sergeant Mom, and Kristen, the military Child Development Center (CDC) was easily and readily available for their children upon returning back to work after maternity leave. For others, however, finding childcare caused significant anxiety.

For one, many servicewomen found themselves on waitlists that were exponentially longer than they had anticipated. For example, Elizabeth, a Navy officer, recalled how her first baby was on the CDC day care waitlist for three years. When she was stationed at the Pentagon, she said she finally got off the waitlist when she had about six months before she was due to transfer. At that point, she said that she'd already established a routine for her son and did not want to disrupt it six months before moving. Similarly, Getoya cited that, "one of the things I was not prepared for and I'm still struggling with is childcare after giving birth." She was advised to sign up for the government childcare as soon as she found out she was pregnant, and did so, thinking it seemed a bit ridiculous. Yet, at the time of our interview, her daughter had just turned ten months old, and they were still on the CDC waitlist. In fact, she said they were on *four* waitlists, and had no idea when they would get in to any of them. Lynn did not know that she needed to get on the waitlist as soon as she knew she was pregnant, so she did not start calling about childcare until she was on maternity leave. She said the CDC had a nine-month waitlist, and other day cares in the area had three- to six-month waitlists. At the last minute, they found a day care with an opening because another servicemember had just received orders to move, so they were fortunate to get childcare before Lynn had to return to work. However, until that point, Lynn said she was "panicking, thinking, 'I'm going to have to take extra leave beyond the twelve weeks because I cannot find day care.'" Being pregnant and recovering from pregnancy can already be physically, emotionally, and mentally taxing, and the additional pressure resulting from the inability to find childcare can significantly exacerbate pregnancy-related stress.

In a couple cases, when the servicewomen could not find care right away, their parents stepped in. This was the case for Clementine, who is a helicopter pilot in the Air Force married to an Air Force pilot. She explained that she was "very, very lucky in that my mom is fully retired and was able to come out and help me with childcare." Getoya also said that as she waited to hear back from the CDC and the four other waitlists, she and her husband flew her mother-in-law in every week to watch her child. As she explained, "at first this was a Monday through Friday kind of thing, and then you'd go home for the weekend, and then we decided 'You know what, two weeks at a time,' and she's loved the quality time, but her marriage . . . ." In this case, Getoya's mother-in-law also had to make sacrifices due to childcare availability issues.

Another issue with childcare is the time day care facilities are open. Many of the servicewomen, including Michelle, Elizabeth, Roxanne, and Clementine commented on how much of the time, day care hours do not accommodate shift workers. For example, Elizabeth explained, "a lot of the people, they don't work nine to five, and civilian day cares aren't structured for people who work shift work." Clementine verified this, explaining that with her shift work, and her husband also in the military and deploying, even the CDC, which is supposed to be childcare to help military families, did not offer hours that would accommodate her schedule. In contrast, Roxanne could have used the extended hours of the CDC (it opened at 6 a.m., and her civilian day care opened at 7 a.m., which was a hardship for her with needing to be at work at 7:30 a.m.), but there was not a spot available.

These stories illuminate another gap that needs to be filled for working mothers in the military. If childcare is not available and/or not available at the times when it is needed (for cases such as shift work), the anxiety and stress it can cause for servicewomen and their families makes it difficult for servicewomen to "have it all." Since servicewomen are likely distracted by the stress of finding childcare, they may not be able to return to work as "mentally fit" as the military hopes per OPNAV 6001.C(209)(a)(2), cited earlier.

PHYSICAL READINESS

Finally, unlike civilian organizations, those who serve in the military are held to physical fitness standards via the Physical Readiness Test

(PRT), and this includes servicewomen who return to work after maternity leave. In recent years, the standards have changed a bit, and servicewomen are given more time before they have to test after the birth of their children. The PRT includes standards for fitness, such as running and push-ups, as well as a body weight requirement based on a person's height. To some, it was not an issue. Kristen, a Navy officer, even turned it into a time to bond with her daughter. She said that once she was able to, she started doing push-ups at home, and then would lay her baby daughter on the floor next to her when doing sit-ups.

Others, however, struggled with the requirements. Elizabeth explained how, even before having children, she'd always been "riding the border on the standards." Therefore, after her first child, she hired a personal trainer to come to her house three times a week at six weeks postpartum to help her get back in shape. Although she said that many in the military would argue she did not have to accrue that extra expense because the military gym offers those services for free, she said if she went to the base, she would want to work, not exercise. After her second child, she never was able to lose all of the weight. As she neared the end of her career, she said she thought, "I can fail it two times. So, in my last two PT tests I failed it. And they're like, 'Oh, don't you care?' I'm like, yeah I care, but for twenty years I would starve myself for two months before the PT test to make weigh in. And then I gained it back and starved and gained and then the babies." Once she knew her retirement timeline, she was able to factor in her PT test failures so they would not tank her career.

Many others expressed anxiety due to the fitness test and expectations to get "back to a weight that the Navy determines" as Magellan stated. Emily, an enlisted Navy servicewoman, explained that she felt that they should be given more time before they were required to test after having a baby. Master Sergeant Mom also expressed, "So, when I'm pregnant, I'm exempted from PT testing, but I *know* that 180 days from the day I give birth, I have to take a PT test. So, I have six months from the day I deliver to go out there and perform like

I did before I had a baby, and that's *hard.*" The person who was the most concerned about the PRT, however, was Natalie, an enlisted servicewomen who ended up having emergency hip surgery shortly after delivering her daughter. In her words, "So, I'm trying to figure out how I'm going to do this. 'Cause I can't even get my weight down as fast as most people because they're able to go run and all this other stuff and I can barely walk. So, trying to figure out that stuff, that's what really worries me. [It's] about getting back to standards." The unique requirements of a career in the military mean that women must work to get back in shape to meet the physical fitness standards if they hope to keep their jobs. This can be overwhelming during a time of healing, lack of sleep, pressure to find childcare, and, in Natalie's case, dealing with an additional health issue.

Meeting physical fitness standards is important for another reason beyond keeping one's job: getting in shape also helps women fit their uniforms again. As Cindy explained, "uniforms definitely put the pressure on you to—not that you can get completely back to your original weight. But, you know, for being motivated not to have to buy more uniforms." As she points out, the uniform serves as an additional motivator to get back in shape quickly because uniforms are expensive, and if a uniform does not fit properly, servicemembers have to purchase ones that do.

THE "CHOICES" OF GOOD WORKING MOTHERS

After having children, many servicewomen found balancing a highly ambitious career and balancing children extremely difficult. Often, they found themselves being asked to choose one over the other. In nearly every conversation about this tension, participants used the rhetoric of choice. The rhetoric of choice implies that servicewomen actually have a choice, and does not take into consideration the ways in which the choice may be constrained. Despite many women feeling a tremendous amount of pressure to take responsibility and act as if nothing changed after they had their children, some voiced dissent from this point of view. Lynn explained how she was told she had to go away for TDY when her child was four months old. She pushed back, citing the policy that stated she was not to be deployed or TDY within the first year after having her baby. Her command responded that she could either do TDY now for a month and a half or it would be tacked on to her six-month deployment once the baby turned one. Because she did not want to be gone for nearly eight months in the second year of her child's life, she "chose" to do TDY when her baby was four months old.

The rhetoric of choice also affords servicewomen agency in a situation they may otherwise feel has taken away their ability to act. For example, Kristen's explanation was populated with the word "choice," as she discussed why she deployed when her daughter was so little:

> It's all personal choice, at least from the officer levels in my community.... So it's a choice, I chose to go to a carrier after I had my daughter, so I deployed for 313 days. So, I missed from like two to three and a half. I was in and out a lot but it was a choice I made to do it because I knew it would be good for my career and she was young enough at that time, I knew she wouldn't remember. So I asked to go to do it kind of early in my career, or earlier than I would have because I knew she wouldn't have that retainment at that point in time. So, I was like, "You know what, I should really go to the carrier now because she's not going to—she has no thought of time, like a week, month, a year means nothing to her in her little brain right now." So I chose to do that; that was a choice I made.

In Kristen's case, it seems that she was attempting to control the narrative in order to avoid the stigma, a common theme when it comes to the rhetoric of choice.[104]

Cindy explained that the reason she was a lieutenant commander for over half her career (not promoting as soon) was "part of the decisions I made as far as the job—well, some of it is you don't have a lot of choices of jobs because of the timing thing. Now, I did pay for that career-wise, but I was fine with that." In Cindy's explanation, she recognizes that some of the decisions were out of her control, such as the timing of events, but she ultimately takes responsibility when it comes to how she responded to poorly timed circumstances. Framing the experience this way reflects how Hays discussed the concept of choice with the good-working-mother identity, "If you are a good mother, you *must* be an intensive one. The only 'choice' involved is whether you *add* the role of paid working woman."[105]

Furthermore, the rhetoric of choice does not take into consideration systemic factors that do not accommodate for dual-career families.[106] Elizabeth noted how the military organization's demands do not support a model with a working mother and father.[107] Echoing this, Paige remembered one woman admiral who had three children, but then qualified that the woman's husband was retired from the Navy and "he was the one who was keeping them together, body and soul."

Michelle and others also talked about how few married women with children there were in the highest ranks. Michelle said she knew of one female O-6 who was married and had one child. Sadie commented that she did not know any female officers above her who had children. Paige elaborated,

> I'm thinking of the women I've known who are senior to me and were two-star and three-star admirals and even four-star admirals—none of them had any children. . . . Some of them are married, but a lot of them married late. In fact, one of the ones I know who made to two stars, she married as a one-star. I mean, it's not that she didn't want it, but she married as a one-star. I know another woman who's a three-star. She's been married forever to the same guy, but they never had any children. I don't know if that was by choice or because she couldn't get pregnant. I don't know. She didn't have any children and she's a great lady and terrific at her job, but she's three stars.

This observation by Paige should not be surprising, given that other scholars, such as Blair-Loy, have found that women who work in male-dominated fields, when compared to their male colleagues or women in other occupations, are far more likely to be unmarried and childless by the "choices" they make.[108]

Others discussed how the health of their children impacted the decisions they made in their careers. Paige explains how she was told she'd be a "shoo-in" for admiral, and was still thinking that was a possibility after having her third child. However, when she found out she was pregnant with her fourth child (an unplanned pregnancy), she said she realized, "I'm just too tired. I can't keep up. I mean, the higher—the energy it takes to be the admiral and the time and the attention versus also having a nine-year-old." So, although she did take some big jobs, like fleet forces, after having her fourth child, she decided that she had a different career trajectory. Throughout all of this, Paige did not blame the military for the tension she felt, but instead attributed it to her own choices. She explained that the military was not "keeping me down, saying, 'Oh, she's got four children. Am I going to let her do that?' but I was limiting myself based on the decisions I was making." Ultimately, she decided it was more important to be home, than to stay at the office two more hours. As Paige was getting close to retirement, she discovered her son had mental illness. She said that "in the Navy, you can't work less." So because she was at the point of retirement, and because she could not work part-time, and because she was tired from her long and intense career in the Navy, she and her husband decided she would retire so she could stay home with her son.

Elsa's son had been born with health issues that caused his urine to go back up to his kidneys. He had to have emergency surgery when he was born and stayed in NICU for two weeks. After the surgery, she had been told that in about one year her son would need multiple surgeries, and possibly a kidney replaced. Two months after her son was born, she received a call that the transfer she had wanted, from aviation to public affairs, was approved. She was so excited, and asked if she could stay in San Diego. She was told she could, but that she was required to go to sea for ten months. She explained that her son had health issues, and asked if there was any way to negotiate, because she could not imagine being out to sea when her baby was in surgery. The detailer told her it was a "take-it-or-leave-it" decision, so she said she chose to leave it, choosing to be with her son.

What can be noted in these narratives is that, in addition to giving servicewomen a sense of control, the emphasis on personal choice also proliferates the rhetoric of responsibilization, wherein servicewomen are relieving the military of any responsibility in their situations, believing that they are solely responsible for the tension they feel between their careers and their families. This is why McCarver argues that the rhetoric of choice is damaging—it gives the impression of choice, free will, and autonomy, but in reality it "employs neoliberal ideas and values to mask a series of narrow scripts, each delineating a limiting and unfavorable 'choice' dangerous to women, feminism, and gender relations in its obfuscation of oppression and patriarchy."[109] Ironically, the very rhetoric of choice employed by servicewomen reinforces the limited options available to them.

In all of the discourses of intensive mothering and good workers, the rhetoric of choice supports the postfeminist notion that McCarver claims "dilutes the meaning of feminism and its relevancy to women's lives, it diverts attention from oppressive social systems and focuses on the individual, avoiding the more difficult to tackle and achieve systemic change necessary in struggles for gender equality."[110] Numerous scholars have noted the connection between postfeminism and choice rhetoric, arguing that it focuses on individuals, rather than systemic issues.[111] As a result, servicewomen end up reinforcing aspects of a constraining culture instead of changing it like the policies attempt to do.

STRUGGLES OF SUPERMOMS

In a time where the rhetoric of choice is emphasized and perpetuated, and is intimately intertwined with the discourses and identities of the good worker, the good mother, and the good working mother, the ultimate identity that emerges for working mothers, and especially the working mothers in the military, is that of the supermom. Douglas and Michaels, as well as O'Brien Hallstein, explain that the ultimate integration of the ideology and rhetoric of choice is the supermom, the mother who can do it all. Many scholars have found that the identity of the supermom is an impossible standard for working mothers, imposed both by society and by women themselves.[112] Cindy, a former Navy officer, explained how the superwoman identity is often a natural development for servicewomen: "As women, especially military women, so we can feel somewhat invincible, like, we've got this; we can do this." Because women can choose to have children and a career, and because they can often be successful at both, the feelings of invincibility create a supermom identity.

The supermom identity has developed in response to a culture that emphasizes women's personal choices to work and have kids, making women ultimately responsible for negotiating the balance between the two parts of their lives.[113] Because women have wanted both—to be mothers and to be good workers—they have found the best way to negotiate the terrain is to work very hard in both areas of their lives to prove they are in many ways invincible and able to do all things. (In contrast, these standards are not applied to men and fathers.) Ultimately, because women enact the role of supermom, it perpetuates and supports, rather than challenges, the belief that this is a reasonable expectation for working mothers. Therefore, although the supermom identity can be very empowering, it can also be very detrimental because of its emphasis on individualism. This means that if, at some point, a woman realizes the difficulty of trying to balance everything, the support needed may not be there.

In one extreme example, Elizabeth recounted how she had severe postpartum depression after her first baby, which she thought had "been exacerbated by the fact that emotionally I had no support other than my husband, who also was transitioning because of his work, and no family around, didn't know the neighbors, didn't know the doctor. I'd step in the shower six times a day so I could cry so no one would hear me, and I didn't want my husband to know what a wreck I was." Elizabeth had moved to Hawaii at eight months pregnant, relocating herself and her husband, and met the doctor who delivered her baby for the first time when she was in the delivery room. After delivery, she suffered from postpartum depression symptoms (PDS), which one in nine mothers in the United States experiences, yet tried to hide it from her husband, essentially "faking it until she made it," as Claudia said most new mothers have to do when they go back to work.[114] The rhetoric of choice that surrounds the supermom identity reinforces the idea that women are to find solutions to their problems, and it absolves the system of any responsibility. In cases like Elizabeth's, this can be dangerous and unnecessary, since there are options to help mothers suffering from PDS.

Furthermore, despite the rhetoric of choice, many servicewomen are obligated to stay in the military—without a choice—because of the choice they made to join it in the first place. Therefore, although the postpartum struggles related to work/life balance may be similar between servicewomen and those in the civilian world, Tanya, a surface warfare officer in the Navy, pointed out how the commitment she made to the military differentiates her from her civilian friends. She explained that "I owe them time, and not because I was home for the pregnancy but because I committed to it and I can't just walk away at this point." She recounted how some of her civilian friends took extended maternity leaves at their jobs, and then decided they were not going to return to work. In contrast, she said, "that's not an option for us. You're going back. You figure out how it all works." Tanya's words reinforce the responsibility of servicewomen to figure out how to balance work and childcare. Hayden and O'Brien Hallstein explained that although understandings and assumptions about women's participation in the public sphere of the workplace have changed, "institutions and family structures have not," so women are basically on their own as they figure out how to meet and balance work and family responsibilities.[115]

RESISTING CULTURAL PRESSURES: (WO)MENTORING

Despite a deep-seated ideology of the intensive good working mother among military women, many voiced resistance to the narrative and sought alternative informal options to navigate the tension, often via mentoring. For example, Roxanne was frustrated by a culture that seemed to ask servicewomen to give up their personal/private lives for their work/public careers. She said,

> So I mean, it's just—[having a baby is] a natural part of life, it's not some strange thing that we do. You shouldn't have to give up a personal part of your life for a job. It's just a job. I know it's a little bit more intense than just like going to the office every day. It affects a lot more of our lives than it does the average civilian. But, it's still a job. And, I'm still allowed to have every other part of my life. I don't think when we sign on the dotted line, we give up everything.

Her discussion highlights the public/private sphere distinction that scholars have noted when studying working mothers. As women continue to enter and promote within the workforce, it becomes more apparent how, as Martin says, "This alleged dichotomy between the public and private spheres of influence is a false distinction."[116] Therefore, although Roxanne desires that the division between the public and private remain, it may not be possible, especially in the military where this distinction is sometimes difficult to maintain because of how the military needs to monitor the health of its members for operational purposes.

Unlike Roxanne, Frida did not realize the need to resist until after she retired. She reflected that now, as a mentor, when servicewomen ask her, "How do you do it or how do I need to do it?" her answers surprise her. She said,

> What I have told these young lieutenants who are trying to figure out how to do it as well, that they don't have to be superwoman and that they don't have to try and prove.... Even the small three weeks

that I've been gone in retirement or leave or whatever, you think there's so much on you and I have so much responsibility and I need to answer this and you're made to feel a little bit like you're the only one that can do it, because the Navy pumps you up that way. "Oh my God. How could we possibly live without you, Frida?" You know what? This organization's been cooking along for 242 years all by itself with way better people than me. And so, I understand the feeling because I've had that feeling of I have to be there or I need to prove it or I don't want anybody to think I'm a slacker. So my advice honestly to these girls is, "Stop. Don't try to do what I did. There's no reason to try and do this superwoman role. Go take your time with your kids. Go. They're giving you this time. The work is still going to be there."

In hindsight, Frida reflects that she should have been easier on herself, and she should have taken the time with her children instead of putting pressure on herself to be superwoman.

Similar to how Frida gives advice to servicewomen, mentoring was very important for many of the participants and served as another form of resistance. Elizabeth mentored Kristen, and told her that they wear four hats: the mom, the wife, the professional, and you. Kristen said it was helpful to have a mentor who had successfully navigated having children in the military, to help her keep things in perspective, and also give her advice on how to approach different aspects of the work-life balance. Likewise, Elsa believed that her experience was "easier than most" because she had a mentor who had a baby the year before and "paved the way for me. And the things that I probably would have felt a lot more guilty for, she would make me feel better about, showing that 'you're not going to be on time for everything, and you're going to have to take a break for you, and remember breastfeeding is for your baby, and you need to do that.'" The advice Elsa received reiterates much of the intensive mothering rhetoric while also giving her permission to ease up on efforts of macho maternity.

Other advice Frida and Paige both gave servicewomen was that the best way to succeed at the work/motherhood tension was to "marry well" or "marry the right person." Because the demands of the job are so significant, especially for women who want to advance and make a career in the military, it is very important to have support at home, someone who can offer some sort of stability. Of course, although Frida and Paige use heteronormative examples, the main point is that there needs to be support at home. Another option that Candee often said she would pitch to servicewomen is the option of the Reserves, because it is a great way for people to have the flexibility they need in their schedules, but still continue to serve their country.

In most of these options, with the exception of Frida advocating for taking full leave, it should be noted that the system does not change, but rather the servicewomen's actions and mindsets do. This reflects Koerber's observation that "individuals might resist certain elements of disciplinary rhetoric, but they never escape the grid of disciplinary power altogether."[117] Ultimately, adhering to responsibilization discourse, the servicewomen changed more than the institution, which will not ultimately result in cultural change.

WHAT NEXT?

After reading the policies and hearing from servicewomen about their efforts to maintain the ideal worker identity, breastfeed their babies for the recommended amount of time, find childcare, and pass the PRT postpartum, three main solutions seem helpful. First, although many of the servicewomen in this chapter seemed to find mentors through their informal networks, there is a need for a more formal mentoring system for pregnant servicewomen in the military. Those who had mentors and were able to ask questions from women who had "been there, done that" as active-duty servicewomen had better experiences, and also found advocates within the hypermasculine organization. Moreover, those mentors who are further along in their careers or are now retired have the gift of hindsight and perspective. However, most of the women who discussed mentoring were officers, and it is unclear if enlisted servicewomen have the same informal mentoring experiences, which is why a more formal (wo)mentoring system seems appropriate.

Additionally, there is a clear need for expanded childcare options for servicemembers, in terms of both availability and hours. Since I conducted the interviews, many Child Development Centers (CDCs) in the military have extended their open hours from twelve to fourteen hours a day, but more work is needed in terms of dual-military, divorced, or single-parent families, as well as other situations that may involve odd hours due to shiftwork and deployment.[118] Additionally, the waitlists need to be taken into consideration, especially if servicewomen who sign up for the waitlist when they are first pregnant still cannot get their child into CDC care by the time the child is two or three years old.

Finally, other ways to break the circuit of discipline may involve servicewomen taking their full maternity leaves, not waiving deferred deployments, asking for non-bathroom locations to pump, and reminding their colleagues of their policy-granted rights as nursing mothers. It is important to note that if servicewomen want the military to adhere to policies, then they, too, should collectively do their part, understanding that they are fighting a systemic issue, not an individual one, and the solution will likely come from a collective effort.

6 Redefining Military Maternity

> When the women are talking about, "Oh well, I went right back to work and deployed in six weeks. And that's what you do when you're in the military." No, it takes someone to step back and say that wasn't right. And we need to change that and be those vocal places. And say that was the military then. And this is the military now.
>
> —Elizabeth

Three years after the image of Air Force servicewomen Christina Luna and Terran Echegoyen-McCabe ignited public conversations about breastfeeding and "proper" use of a military uniform, more photos of servicewomen breastfeeding in uniform emerged. In March 2015, Staff Sergeant Jonea Cunico, an aircraft electrical and environmental specialist in the Air Force Reserves, was photographed breastfeeding her fourteen-month-old son while in uniform (see figure 6.1). In this image, Cunico is standing against a plain light gray background, presumably in a photo studio. She is wearing a combat uniform and combat boots while holding her child across her body, his head at her left breast, and his hips by her right hip. Her shirt is slightly lifted to accommodate breastfeeding, but little of her skin is shown, as her son covers where her shirt is absent. She makes eye contact with the camera, and has a confident, expression.

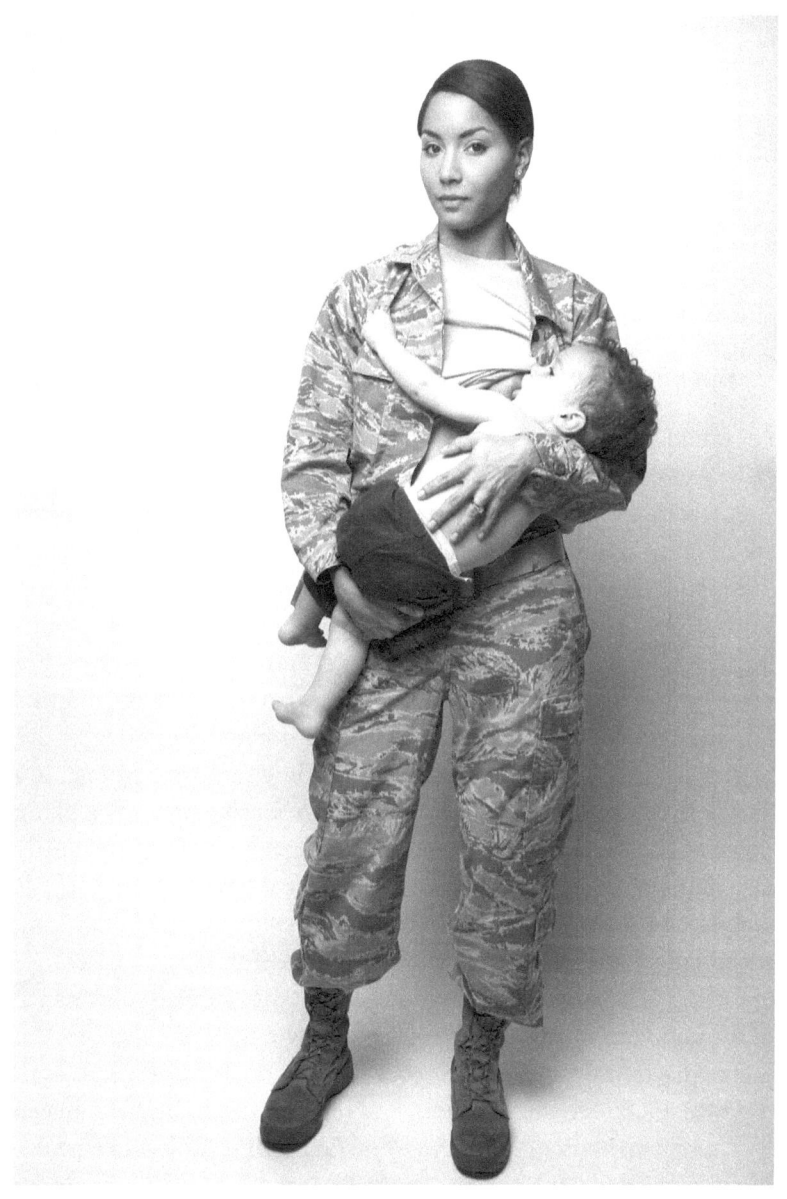

Figure 6.1. Staff Sgt. Jonea Cunico, pictured in 2015 breastfeeding her son. Image used with permission of Jade Beall Photography.

Robyn Roche-Paull, founder of Breastfeeding in Combat Boots, promoted the photograph, taken by Jade Beall, on her website,

> This photo is more than just that of a mother breastfeeding her child. This photo is more than just that of a member of the Air Force Reserves breastfeeding her toddler in uniform. This is a photo that shows us what motherhood in the military looks like. This photo shows us a mother who is both beautiful and strong. This photo shows us a mother who is both a nurturer and a fighter. This photo shows us a mother who is a protector of both her child and her country. This photo shows us a mother who wears her uniform with honor and professionalism while giving her child the very best start in life.[1]

Beall took this photo as part of her project of capturing what she calls "sheros" (she + heros).[2]

A few months later, in September 2015, photographer Tara Ruby took pictures of a group of servicewomen breastfeeding in uniform (figure 6.2). This image resembles the one of Ecegoyen-McCabe and Luna in that it is also taken outside in a field or park. The sun is shining, the blue sky has a few wispy clouds, and ten servicewomen are pictured in the center of the image in combat camouflage uniforms holding their children to their breasts to nurse them. Their entire bodies are visible. Five women are standing, and five women are either sitting or kneeling in front of them. Each woman is looking down at her child, and each is also wearing a hat, effectively mostly or completely covering their faces, creating a type of anonymity, or feeling that these women represent all nursing mothers in uniform. Although all are breastfeeding, there is no visible cleavage. Because of the lack of cleavage, the size of the group, the zoomed-out distance of the photograph, and the use of hats to cover the women's faces, the image places the focus on the modest act of breastfeeding babies in uniform, likely evoking a less visceral response than the 2012 image.

This group photograph was part of Tara Ruby's project to normalize breastfeeding and decorate the walls of the new nursing room for the Army Base at Fort Bliss in El Paso, Texas.[3] Because research finds that exposure to breastfeeding helps increase women's self-efficacy,

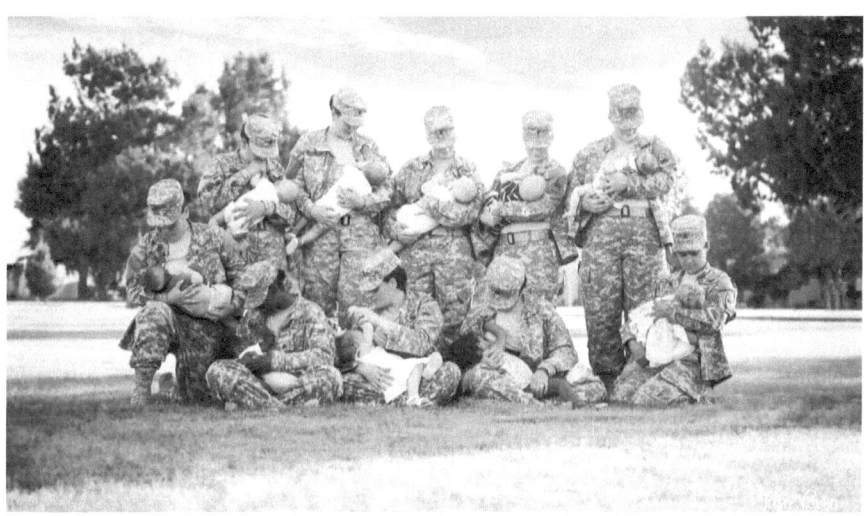

Figure 6.2. Servicewomen breastfeeding in uniform in 2015. Image used with permission of Tara Ruby Photography, www.tararuby.com.

if servicewomen see images of their peers and colleagues breastfeeding in uniform, something that has not been discussed much publicly until recently, they may realize that it is also an option for them.[4]

In contrast to the 2012 image—where the servicewomen and photograph were met with significant resistance and were reprimanded by the Air Force for inappropriate use of the uniform to promote a cause—the images taken by Beall and Ruby were approved by the Air Force and the Army, respectively.[5] Almost a year later, another photo shoot of active-duty servicewomen breastfeeding in uniform took place in Washington, D.C., as part of the official "Normalize Breastfeeding" project by photographer Vanessa Simmons.[6] The increase in images of servicewomen breastfeeding in uniform, and the decrease in resistance from the public and the military may be evidence of progress in, acceptance of, and support for servicewomen's maternity experiences.

In fact, in recent years there has been an evolution of military maternity and parental policy changes. The interviews for this project concluded in early 2017, eighteen months after the Navy announced the eighteen-week maternity leave policy, and one year after all military maternity policies were changed to twelve weeks of leave for the birth mothers in an effort to ensure all military maternity policies were consistent across the services. Those DoD-wide maternity leave policy changes have been credited as stimuli for more recent changes related to pregnancy and parenthood.[7]

In addition to the so-called gender-neutral changes in uniforms discussed in chapter 2, the language used in policies has moved toward a more gender-neutral tone, as well. For example, in the early Instructions for the Navy, OPNAVINST 6000.1A (1989), OPNAVINST 6000.1B (2003), and OPNAVINST 6000.1C (2007), the language in the policies referred to "pregnant servicewomen."[8] In all of these documents, pregnant servicewomen were granted forty-two days of convalescent leave. The use of "convalescence" instead of "maternity" leave in some ways serves to frame servicewomen's leave as gender-neutral; however, it can also be argued that the use of this term implies that pregnancy is a disability or illness to be cured. More discussion on this type of rhetoric was covered in chapter 4, but it is worth repeating that pregnancy is often pathologized, as if it is something to be cured or something that is disabling, instead of a natural part of human life.[9]

With the newest Instructions, OPNAVINST 6000.1D, released in March 2018, there is a notable language change. Instead of *servicewomen* the term *service members* is used. This change is part of a larger cultural shift in the military to avoid using gendered language when referring to military personnel. For example, looking at policies in the Army, one can note that they refer to "Soldiers who want to breastfeed."[10] In the Air Force, women are referred to as "personnel who are pregnant," "AF members who are breastfeeding or pumping," and also "Airmen who are breastfeeding" ("airmen" is considered a gender-neutral term).[11] In fact, the Marine Corps stand out as still using the term *servicewomen*, although the language "pregnant Marine" is also used.

Yet research has shown that attempting to mask or minimize "gender differences with gender-neutral language does not, as a strategy, appear to be working as a means for advancing gender equality."[12] What Smithson and Stokoe found in their research of maternity leave in a male-dominated organization was that so-called "genderblind" terms did not change widespread assumptions about events and concepts often linked to women. In the case of the military, this is even more evident, as a tension is present when using gender-neutral language in that "pregnant" is juxtaposed with a neutral sex. Smithson and Stokoe discovered, then, that "language change without corresponding culture change is bound to fail."[13] In fact, researchers have found that even with the implementation of gender-fair language, gender stereotyping still exists, because people associate certain roles in society with certain genders.[14]

Another change that occurred with the release of OPNAVINST 6000.1D was from the term *convalescent leave* to *maternity leave*. This is interesting, especially since convalescent leave is a more neutral term. In essence, the Navy swapped one gendered and one gender-neutral term for another. Language changed from "servicewomen" receiving "convalescent leave" to "service members" receiving "maternity leave." This means that any assumptions that the Navy was perhaps switching to the use of a gender-blind sex were in efforts to recognize the spectrum of sexualities and possibilities within those sexualities may not be the case. Because *maternity leave* is a very gendered term (many of the current debates circulate around *maternity* versus *parental* leave and the implications of the different terms), gender is still very much part of the discussion around maternity in the military.

The most dramatic policy change occurred DoD-wide in June 2018, when the undersecretary of defense issued a memo laying out new maternity and parental leave policies in the cases of birth or adoption of children.[15] Ultimately, this new policy combines the previous parenting policies into one, and replaced the current adoption, maternity, and paternity leaves, as well as caregiver designations.[16] In this document, the new language is "maternity convalescent leave," combining previous iterations.[17] The new policy, however also includes two other types of leave that were not previously included in other policies. One is the Primary Caregiver Leave (PCL) and the other is Secondary Caregiver Leave (SCL). Previously, there was maternity leave of forty-two days (6 weeks) or eighty-four days (twelve weeks) and in 2007 the first implementation of paternity leave of ten consecutive days (as long as the man was married to the baby's mother). Now, instead, there is "Parental Leave for Members of the Armed Forces" (although many people still use parental, paternity, and secondary caregiver leave synonymously). Since June 2018, Maternity Convalescent leave is six weeks given to the birthparent after a "qualifying event." This is important to note, as it reverts back to the policies in place prior to Ash Carter's January 2016 announcement of twelve weeks of nonchargeable leave for birthmothers. Under the 2018 policy, designated primary caregivers may take an additional six weeks within the first year of the birth of their child. This is often the mother. Secondary caregivers are to be given up to twenty-one days of leave, depending on the branch of the military. Secondary caregivers are often the fathers. This is a significant increase from previous paternity leave policies, which gave fathers (who are married to birth mothers) ten consecutive days of paternity leave. However, each branch is allowed to decide how much leave they will give servicemembers, and, as such, the Air Force and Coast Guard are granting the full twenty-one-day leave, whereas the Navy and Marine Corps are giving fourteen days.[18]

Many have applauded the gender-neutral language used in the new policy and the flexibility it offers, because the gender-neutral designation of PCL and SCL allows for inclusion of diverse types of families, such as dual-military, single parents, same-sex parents, transgender parents, and unmarried parents.[19] The new policy challenges the relentless expectation "that mothers are more responsible for family life than are fathers."[20] With the new policy, if a father is considered the primary caregiver, he may now be eligible for up to six weeks of leave within the first year of the child's life. The mother, if designated the secondary caregiver, would get only six weeks (instead of twelve). By making these changes, the military is moving away from the assumption that women are and/or should be the primary caregivers, an assumption that was built in to previous policies. While it may still be accurate for most people, the flexibility offered in the new policy is a good step.[21]

In addition to maternity policy changes, in 2012, the Army announced that it was going to start testing and implementing ACU-A uniforms, or "Army Combat Uniform—Alternate." The uniform has narrower shoulders, elastic waist, tapered waist, more spacious hips and seat areas and was originally part of a female-only approved uniform.[22] However, the Army approved the uniform as unisex, instead of female-only, so that male soldiers who have smaller statures may also wear them. Ultimately, the Defense Advisory Committee to Women in the Services (DACOWITS) argued that a female-only uniform would draw "unwarranted attention to gender differences," which is why it was labeled as a unisex alternate uniform. Of course, although this gender-neutral language is nice in theory, there still are material realities like maternity that require different uniforms, as discussed in chapter 4, which, according to the servicewomen who wear them, are so poorly designed that they make women feel like they stand out more than they should and look more unprofessional than is necessary.

REJECTING MACHO MATERNITY

I began this book by asking about the type of pregnancy culture that is constructed in the military and the ways that servicewomen respond to this culture. I also asked what the consequences of these responses are. Throughout these chapters, it has become evident that military policies, procedures, language, culture, uniforms, and more frame pregnancy as problematic, even if on paper the policies appear to accommodate pregnancy. Pregnancy continues to be constructed as an inconvenience, as making the servicewomen appear weak and incapable, and as a way to get out of required duties.

I found that servicewomen respond to these discourses that frame pregnancy as a problem by participating in and/or advocating for hyperplanning and performing macho maternity (leave). By doing this, servicewomen are engaging in micropractices that contribute to discourses of responsibilization, or intense individual responsibility, when it comes to pregnancy and parenthood. Despite some participants voicing resistance to hyperplanning (because fertility is not always able to be planned or because women want to have agency when it comes to pregnancy, for example), the concept of "appropriate timing" of pregnancies still exists, and is often supported by servicewomen themselves. Likewise, although many of the servicewomen said that they often tell other pregnant servicewomen that they do not have to try to be superwoman and should take advantage of the rest given to them when pregnant, many of them refused to do this themselves. As a result, a loop is created—a circuit of discipline—in which servicewomen's discourses and performances reinforce problematic responsibilization rhetorics.

As I stated in the introduction, these discourses are not limited to the military and servicewomen. For example, Anne-Marie Slaughter, the current president and CEO of New America, challenged the idea that women have complete control over how they sequence their careers and family planning, arguing "the problem is not with women, but with *work*."[23] In contrast to Slaughter, other powerful women exhibit and perpetuate the concept of macho maternity discussed in previous chapters. For instance, prominent businesswoman Marissa Mayer, the CEO of Yahoo, took minimal maternity leave. Sheryl Sandberg, COO of Facebook, emphasized the idea of women "leaning in" at work. Although both of these women, like many of the servicewomen interviewed for this book, were attempting to "make it in a man's world," they simultaneously contributed to the problematic discourses that surround pregnancy and motherhood in society, therefore participating in the proliferation of the double bind in which many of the servicewomen, and likely many working women in general, find themselves. As Frida explained in chapter 4, she did not want to be treated any differently than her non-pregnant self or male colleagues when she was pregnant until she "absolutely did." But at that point, it was difficult to backtrack and ask to take advantage of the accommodations.

A significant problem with advocating for macho maternity and hyperplanning is that instead of challenging and changing cultural discourses about pregnancy, work, and working mothers, they reinforce traditional gender and cultural scripts that support the status quo. The status quo continues to be that working men—who historically have not been hindered by childcare or needed at home—are the standard, the neutral, and that all other workers must become like them. The current scripts that people are following about what it means to be the ideal service member are antiquated and rely on the model of the male breadwinner. This model is not as applicable today, and, as many of the servicewomen I interviewed explained, *they* are the breadwinners in their families now. The problem with this is that much of the responsibility for children-related items is still placed on mothers.[24] This does not mean that fathers do not want to be involved; it means that the discourses surrounding parenthood must change.

For example, Elizabeth discussed the difficulty she had with the current culture in the military: "But the fact that some old white guy who's in his fifties or sixties who has a wonderful woman who's given up everything to be the military wife, typically if they're at that rank—God bless them all—but if you have support of someone at home who has dedicated everything to support your family—well, women usually don't have that, and I'm a working woman with a working husband, and we want a family, and the demands of the organization aren't structured to support that." Similar sentiments have been shared about working in higher education as a professor, where "job descriptions and performance expectations are built on the presumption of a full-time home-based (female) caregiver and homemaker whose job is to ensure the achievements of the full-time (male) academic's career."[25] Furthermore, similar to the military, scholars Townsley and Broadfoot, as well as others, have found that in higher education "the existence of a family-friendly policy does not necessarily mean it will be utilized," much like the findings in this book.[26]

Despite all the pressure related to macho maternity, toward the end of 2018, there came to be what some called the "post–Lean In" moment—essentially women who had embraced the concepts Sandberg promoted in *Lean In* were now rejecting them because of the way that it "placed so much responsibility for success on individual women rather than the societal structures around them."[27] What's more, there has not been much of a change in U.S. companies' family leave programs since the Lean In movement started. As one self-described "former Lean In evangelist" explained, some of the Lean In mentality allowed women to blame themselves for not getting promoted instead of looking at structural inequities. And she pushed even further, explaining that it is "not just saying, 'Oh, if we had paid family leave, everything would be better.' It's so much more than that."[28]

Indeed, this is what the research in this book found. The military has one of the most generous maternity and parental leave policies, and the policies continue to evolve. Their health insurance covers labor and delivery at 100 percent and servicewomen only have to pay for their meals in the hospital. Hospital-grade pumps are provided for free via servicewomen's insurance. Yet, despite these, and other, benefits, servicewomen are still struggling to maintain a work-life balance in the military, and many of them continue to leave in order to try to find that balance in the civilian sector.

Rosa Brooks, a Georgetown University law professor, further discussed the problems with leaning in and macho maternity when combined with intensive mothering, explaining that both require ubiquity—being available via email for work 24/7 as well as being more involved than ever in children's lives and scheduling. This ubiquity affects women more than men. As she states, "And as long as women are the ones doing more of the housework and childcare, women will be disproportionately hurt when both workplace expectations and parenting expectations require ubiquity. They'll continue to do what too many talented women already do: Just as they're on the verge of achieving workplace leadership positions, they'll start dropping out."[29] This is what many of the servicewomen in this book discussed. Mae, a Navy officer who was deeply committed to the military and very supportive of its policies, was leaving due to the difficulty of balancing her work and life because of deployment schedules.

One answer to this, that Brooks gives, is to

> challenge the assumption that more is always better, and the assumption that men don't suffer as much as women when they're exhausted and have no time for family or fun. And we need to challenge those assumptions wherever we find them, both in the workplace and in the family.... We need to fight for our right to lean out, and we need to do it together, girls. If we're going to fight the culture of workplace ubiquity, and the parallel and equally-pernicious culture of intensive parenting, we need to do it together—and we need to bring our husbands and boyfriends and male colleagues along, too. They need to lean out in solidarity, for their own sake as well as ours. Women of the world, recline![30]

Yet, how do we "recline"? How can servicewomen and servicemen challenge the assumptions about maternity in the military and start really changing the culture?

Elizabeth said that she was asked a similar question by the admiral in charge of her office before she left her tour there. She had been frustrated because she felt that during Women's History Month, the things the military was doing felt like tokenism. Her admiral countered her anger by saying, "These are great things. Why are you getting so mad?" Her reply was, "It's not about giving me a year off to be with my kid, although that's nice. It's not going to change the culture. You want to make a change? Quit scheduling meetings at four in the afternoon and expecting someone at eight o'clock in the morning to have answers to the questions you asked at the meeting. Quit expecting people to be here all the time. Allow people to work from home and telecommute. Be more flexible. When you've done that, I will believe that you are an inclusive culture." As I said in the introduction, the voices of servicewomen like Elizabeth who are experiencing maternity in the military are likely the best sources of suggestions as to how the culture can change in a way that makes pregnancy, maternity, and parenthood less of a stigma. They may also have suggestions that will help with the retention of women.

MOVING TOWARD CULTURAL AND SYSTEMIC CHANGE

Approximately 16 percent of active-duty U.S. military forces are women, and the number is growing. Yet women are still underrepresented at the highest ranks, and those who make it that far rarely have children.[31] Nearly 40% of all children of active-duty servicemembers are five years old and younger, which indicates that many servicemembers leave the military while their kids are still young.[32] In fact, despite exemplary maternity policies by U.S. standards, the military's retention of women is still low. To gain perspective on these statistics, I examined the U.S. military's maternity policies, comparing what is said in writing to what is being experienced by servicewomen. It quickly became apparent that the main issues are cultural and systemic, rooted in ideals of military hypermasculinity.

One of the main arguments that undergirds most of the discrimination that servicewomen experience (and the pressure that they put on themselves) is that pregnant women cannot deploy, and that women who have had a baby in the last year cannot be deployed, therefore making them unavailable for the same types of roles in which men and nonpregnant women can serve. If this type of thinking continues, wherein the military's main focus is only on the availability of *bodies* and not on the minds, experiences, and diverse ideas that women of childbearing age can bring to the armed forces, then the answer may be that the military simply stop allowing women to join. If the belief that all women should be able to completely control their fertility or else must completely abstain from sex, despite the fact that their male counterparts are not held to such standards due to their biology, then the military should stop allowing women to join. If women are to be held to moving standards when it comes to their pregnancy planning—for example, being told to have babies when they are on shore duty, and planning accordingly only to have the military's timeline change at the last minute after the servicewomen are already pregnant—then women should not be allowed to join the military.

Yet I do not think the military's intention or desire is to rid the armed forces of women—as can be evidenced by its increasing amount of family- and maternity-friendly policies, and Mabus's statement cited earlier in this book that he wants to see women comprise twenty-five percent of the Navy in the next five years. If the military's desire is to keep recruiting and retaining women, as its leaders often publicly advocate, it needs to start holding itself accountable to its own policies, and actively promoting the belief that "a more diverse force is a stronger force."[33] This means that military members are seen as more than just bodies, and that having women in the military—even if they are unable to serve in certain capacities for short periods of time due to pregnancy—is still more valuable than not having them serve at all. Yet, how can these changes happen culturally, in conjunction with policy? Drawing from my interviews with servicewomen, I want to use the remaining pages to offer some suggestions about where systemic and cultural changes may start.

First, despite being granted a significant amount of maternity leave, many servicewomen were not taking all of it due to guilt that their coworkers were having to do their work while they were gone. Therefore, many women cut their maternity leaves short, and/or worked from home while they were supposed to be recovering from labor and delivery, bonding with their babies, and establishing a breastfeeding routine, if desired. Women (and men) need to take the leave that is granted to them. If they do not, and/or if the culture continues to be one where it is admirable to come back to work earlier than required—the culture of the industrious American warrior discussed in chapter 5—the circuit of discipline is perpetuated, and the culture will never change. Indeed, it is this very culture and attitude that contributes to why many men in the military and elsewhere often refuse parental leave.

Second, despite having their labor and delivery hospital care covered at 100 percent, many servicewomen felt that their overall health care was subpar because of a lack of continuity of care as well as a lack of agency on their part when it came to choosing their providers. Allowing, or even requiring, servicewomen to see OB/GYNs and/or midwives during their pregnancy and postpartum appointments is the first step, since some said they were required to see GPs for their maternity care. Additionally, seeing *the same* caregivers throughout their pregnancy experiences will also help with pregnancy and postpartum satisfaction and comfort. Finally, giving servicewomen *options* as to who they will see for their doctors allows servicewomen agency and contributes to making maternity a more comfortable, personable, and positive experience.

Third, many servicewomen reported feeling like they had no privacy or personal lives because of the requirement to share with their command as soon as they found out they were pregnant. This led servicewomen in some cases to keep their pregnancies hidden, potentially putting their pregnancies at risk, and also disrupting plans for their replacements while they were out due to pregnancy or maternity leave. Rather than helping servicewomen, these policies in some ways hurt servicewomen and the military more. Thankfully, it appears that the Navy is listening to feedback regarding its policies.

For example, as of January 2019, "Service Members who think they may be pregnant are responsible for promptly confirming pregnancy through testing by appropriate medical providers and informing their COs, as appropriate."[34] This is a significant departure from the previous iteration of the policy, which required servicewomen to "notify their CO or officer in charge (OIC) of a pregnancy as soon as possible, but no later than two weeks after diagnosis."[35] The reason for the change in rules, as is stated on the Navy's Pregnancy and Parenthood webpage, is to allow "Service members to maintain privacy and determine the viability of the pregnancy."[36] Making changes like these responds to servicewomen's statements that there is little to no privacy in the military, especially for pregnant servicewomen, who feel like their pregnancy is treated as a "medicalized condition" instead of one of the most "joyous occasions in your personal life," as Tanya, a Navy officer, referred to it.

Fourth, better availability of childcare is needed. This is not a new problem; it is an ongoing cultural problem, and it extends beyond the military. Schwartz said over two decades ago that "the capacity of working mothers to function effectively and without interruption depends on the availability of good, affordable child care."[37] This is still true. If mothers are anxious or distracted about their childcare situation, it will be more difficult for them to focus on work, and they will likely be more difficult to retain. Better options, longer hours, and more availability would be a great start for military mothers and families.

Fifth, (wo)mentoring is needed. Servicewomen need to have support from other women who have "been there, done that" and learned from their mistakes. As I noted in the previous chapter, there is a need for (wo)mentoring in the military when it comes to maternity experiences. Many of the women interviewed for this project were able to find mentors, but not all of them. For many years it has been recognized by other institutions that women, who are often disadvantaged simply for being women, benefit from workplace mentors. This is especially true in the military.[38]

One reason so many women may be leaving is because they do not have mentors at the higher ranks and/or they do not see anyone serving in the higher ranks who is balancing motherhood and a military career. Sadie discussed how rare it is to see women make it to the top ranks as a Navy pilot. She reflected,

> I never had any female senior officers as professional mentors, unfortunately, until I got into the Reserves because there's just so few in aviation, so I didn't know any officers above me that had children.... So, there was one female officer that was lieutenant commander when I was in the squadron, but she was divorced, you know, not wanting kids, and then there was another officer and she was newly married and, you know, she was on one of her sea tours, and so not a lot of people professionally that I talked to about getting pregnant.

When there are few women in the top ranks who have experienced pregnancy, it is not surprising that retention of servicewomen who have children is low.

Yet, it should be noted that while this predominantly affects servicewomen, since they are the ones who physically carry and birth the babies, work-life balance affects men, as well. As a junior-level officer, Candee went to the retirement ceremony of a warrant officer (someone who enlisted and then was commissioned as an officer). He had served about thirty years, and at the ceremony, he stood up and addressed the gathering.

> He held up a piece of paper and it was two-sided, and it's what we call the DD-214, and it's basically your record of service. And he got kind of somber, and he said, "Guess what? This is it, ladies and gentlemen." It was a two-sided sheet of paper, and he said, "What this paper doesn't say, and I want you all to be aware of today, is nineteen birthdays missed, fifteen anniversaries missed. I missed the birth of my third child," dah-dah-dah-dah, and he went through his list of—and I don't think it was regrets. It was just, "Be mindful of the fact that when your time comes to transition, this is it. It's your pension, your benefits, and a piece of paper, and don't let the door hit you on the way out." So it just was another one of those kind of pivotal moments

where you're like, "Okay, good, I need to keep that in mind, that no matter how much they need me or want me, there's other people who are equally deserving of my time and attention."

For Candee, this speech in many ways served as advice from a mentor—helping her put her career and family priorities into perspective.

Sixth, more admirals and supervisors should be asking servicewomen for their thoughts regarding policies and procedures, like Elizabeth's did. Instead of assuming that changing policies was the end-all to accommodate women's needs, Elizabeth voiced concerns over when meetings were scheduled. Scheduling meetings at times that take into consideration working parents' schedules (pick up times from childcare, inability to work at night if they are taking care of children, etc.) can contribute to a more positive experience, and also allow servicemembers, and especially pregnant and parenting servicewomen, to perform at their best levels.

To conclude, there is much work yet to be done when it comes to maternity policies and the culture surrounding maternity, both in the U.S. military and in general U.S. society. Examining the military, which has some of the most generous policies, is a great place to start, with hopes that its policies will influence those in the civilian sector and that, in the not-so-distant-future, pregnant women and working mothers will not be viewed as problematic or as inconveniences, but as important contributors in the workplace. The research in the preceding pages also raises other topics that can be discussed in addition to what has been covered in this book. To start by focusing on this one sphere—women in the military having babies—we can then extend our conversation to related occupations, ones that emphasize hyperplanning, macho maternity, and/or are physically demanding (including, but not limited to, firefighters, academics, law enforcement, and corporate America).[39]

Ultimately, by listening to servicewomen's maternity stories and analyzing their experiences alongside military maternity policies, the reasons for the disconnect between policy and culture became more evident. Changing policies will not result in the dramatic changes that the policies seem to support without addressing the deep-seated cultural ideologies rooted in hypermasculinity, and without listening to servicewomen's voices. I began this book by arguing that we should look at social problems as rhetorical problems and try to find rhetorical correctives that might be put in place in addition to the policy correctives. A good way to start this process is to push back on understandings of what it means to be a good service member, or, similar to Elizabeth's quote in the opening of this chapter, what does it mean to be a good servicemember *today*? Expanding this understanding could have a significant impact in U.S. military maternity culture and beyond.

APPENDIX A **Research Participants: Demographics**

Due to the locations of the participants, most interviews were held virtually via Skype or FaceTime. In some cases, because of a poor connection or other factors, the interview was conducted over the phone, or, in one case, via email (see appendix B). I used semi-structured interview questions for the interviews, which averaged forty-five minutes. Servicewomen picked or were given a pseudonym for anonymity, based on preference.

Table A.1   Demographic Information for Interview Participants

	Enlisted Interviewees (2013)	Officer Interviewees (2016–2017)
Age range	22 to 42; average age of 32 years old	28 to 51, average age of 37 years old
Marital status	• Single: 3 • Married: 5 • Divorced: 4 • Separated: 1	• Single: 0 • Married: 17 • Divorced: 0 • Separated: 1
Branch	• Army: 1 • Air Force: 3 • Navy: 9	• Air Force: 3 • Navy: 15
Rank at time of pregnancy	E-4 (junior enlisted) to E-8 (chief)	O-3 (Navy lieutenant/Air Force captain) to O-4 (Navy lieutenant commander/Air Force major)
Service	3–20 years	5–26 years active duty (not including military academy time)
Ethnicity (self-identified)	• Caucasian: 7 • African American: 3 • Mexican/Guatemalan: 1 • Asian/Filipina: 1 • Native American: 1	• Caucasian: 16 • Black/White/Native American: 1 • Hispanic: 1
Pregnancy planning	• Planned: 6 • Unplanned: 7	• Planned: 34 • Unplanned: 7
Children's ages	2.5 months–11 years old at the time of the interviews	4 months–23 years old at the time of the interviews (plus two pregnant at time of interviews)
Location of participants (at time of interview)	• US (southwest, western, southern, and southeast) • Japan • United Kingdom	All were located in the continental United States

APPENDIX B Profiles: Enlisted Servicewomen

The descriptions below apply to the servicewomen at the time of the interviews and are arranged in chronological order based on the days of each interview.

• JOANNA • AUGUST 3, 2013 • UTAH • IN PERSON • ARMY

Joanna is a veteran who had reached the rank of E-7. A forty-two-year-old Caucasian divorced mother of two boys, ages nine and eleven, she is laid back, candid, and laughs easily. Both of her pregnancies were planned.

• MAGELLAN • AUGUST 28, 2013 • NEVADA • SKYPE • NAVY

Magellan is a friendly and forthright thirty-nine-year-old single Caucasian mother of an eleven-year-old daughter. She was 407 days away from being able to retire and begin working in the civilian sector. Her pregnancy was unplanned.

- MASTER SERGEANT MOM • SEPTEMBER 17, 2013
- UNITED KINGDOM • SKYPE • AIR FORCE

Master Sergeant Mom is a thirty-five-year-old Caucasian mother of two daughters, ages six and four. Recently divorced, she was an E-7. She is knowledgeable and talkative, and speaks rapidly, eager to share her experience with others. She recently earned a master's degree in public administration. Both of her pregnancies were planned.

- IVETTE • SEPTEMBER 22, 2013 • TEXAS • FACETIME
- AIR FORCE

Ivette was a twenty-nine-year-old married mother of two children: an eight-year-old and an almost-two-year-old. She was no longer in the Air Force, but was still in the Air National Guard and was hoping to get back to active duty in the summer of 2014. When she left the Air Force, she was an E-5. She identified her ethnicity as Mexican/Guatemalan. Both of her pregnancies were planned.

- SAMANTHA • OCTOBER 13, 2013 • EAST COAST
- SKYPE • NAVY

Samantha had a five-year-old son at the time of our interview and was separated from her son's father. She is a matter-of-fact Caucasian twenty-five-year-old E-5. Her pregnancy was unplanned.

- JULES • OCTOBER 13, 2013 • EAST COAST • SKYPE • NAVY

Jules was an E-5 servicewoman who had served for six years. She was a twenty-four-year-old Caucasian mother of two, who had recently separated from her children's father. Despite frustrating circumstances surrounding her second pregnancy, she is positive, informed, and direct. Both of her pregnancies were unplanned.

- EMILY • OCTOBER 13–14, 2013 • UNKNOWN
- EMAIL • NAVY

Emily was unable to Skype or talk on the phone, so multiple emails were exchanged with questions and answers. At the time of communication, she was an E-6. She was a married Caucasian thirty-year-old mother of two children, one who was four years old, and the other who was eight months old. Both of her pregnancies were planned.

• JADA • OCTOBER 14, 2013 • MISSISSIPPI • SKYPE • NAVY

Jada was a married African American mother of three children, ages twelve, ten, and two. She is straightforward and well informed. At the time of the interview was ranked an E-7 chief. Her husband was about to retire from the Navy, and she was still planning on serving. Her first pregnancy was unplanned, and the other two were planned.

• MARY • OCTOBER 17, 2013 • CALIFORNIA • SKYPE • NAVY

Mary was a thirty-seven-year-old divorced Native American veteran who had reached the rank of E-6 after serving for almost eighteen years. She is friendly and open. She had three unplanned pregnancies that all resulted in miscarriages.

• ARIEL • OCTOBER 21, 2013 • CALIFORNIA • SKYPE • NAVY

A confident forty-year-old Caucasian E-8 servicewoman at the time of the interview, Ariel had almost served twenty-two years. Her son was seventeen months old, and she also had two stepchildren, ages six and sixteen, with her husband. Her pregnancy was planned.

• SYDNEY • OCTOBER 22, 2013 • CALIFORNIA
• SKYPE • NAVY

Sydney was a soft-spoken, twenty-two-year-old African American E-4 sailor at the time of our interview. She had been in the Navy for three years, and her baby was seven months old. She was single. Her pregnancy was unplanned.

• NATALIE • OCTOBER 26, 2013 • WEST COAST
• SKYPE • NAVY

Natalie was a quiet African American mother of a three-month-old daughter. She was a twenty-six-year-old E-5 at the time of the interview. She had been in the Navy for three years and was single, although she was engaged to the father of her baby. Her pregnancy was unplanned.

- CLARISSA • OCTOBER–NOVEMBER, 2013 • CALIFORNIA
- EMAIL • AIR FORCE

Clarissa communicated via email since the government shutdown in October 2013 made it difficult for her to find time to be able to Skype. She was an E-5 with three children, ages twelve, six, and five. She was a married thirty-four-year-old who identified herself as Asian/Filipino.

APPENDIX C Profiles: Female Officers

The descriptions below apply to the servicewomen at the time of the interviews and are arranged in chronological order based on the days of each interview.

- ELIZABETH • APRIL 6, 2016 • CALIFORNIA • SKYPE • NAVY

Elizabeth is a Caucasian, married, forty-four-year-old veteran. She served as an officer for twenty years, and retired from the military ranked as a commander (O-5). She has two children, a daughter who is eleven years old and a son who is eight years old. She planned her first pregnancy and the second one was a surprise. Elizabeth is proactive, well-informed, friendly, and matter-of-fact. She was pursuing her PhD in organizational communication at the time of the interview. Her husband was not in the military. Elizabeth was a main recruiter for this project and is highly regarded among many of the women in this study.

- MIRANDA • APRIL 6, 2016 • OHIO • PHONE • NAVY

Miranda has served fifteen years, first as a surface warfare officer (SWO) and then as a public affairs officer (PAO). In 2012 she transitioned to be a reservist so that she could keep the military insurance without such an intense military schedule. The insurance is especially important, since her third child was born with cystic fibrosis. She has four children—ages nine, six, four, and one. All her pregnancies were planned, and she experienced a miscarriage between her first two children. Her husband did not serve in the military. Miranda is a Caucasian lieutenant commander (O-4). She is thirty-seven years old and is very open and friendly.

- MICHELLE • APRIL 7, 2016 • SOUTH DAKOTA
- SKYPE • NAVY

Michelle is part of a dual-military marriage—she recently retired as an O-5 (commander) naval intelligence officer and her husband is an O-6 (captain) in the Air Force. Part of her retirement was prompted by her inability to co-locate with her husband as they both moved up in rank. At age forty-five, she had served twenty-one years in the Navy, and had two children, a ten-year-old son (she had him as an O-4) and a seven-year-old daughter (who was born when she was an O-5). Her son was in the same room as her in the beginning of the interview because a package had arrived in the mail and it was his birthday. He was only present for the first five minutes. Michelle is Caucasian and a very persistent and dedicated woman, mother, and spouse with a lot of grit. Both of Michelle's pregnancies were planned.

- CINDY • APRIL 8, 2016 • WASHINGTON, D.C.
- PHONE • NAVY

A retired lieutenant commander (O-4), Cindy served in the military for twenty years. At age forty-three, she is a very fast talker, well informed, and eager to talk about her experience as a pregnant servicewoman as well as an active-duty mother. Cindy grew up in a military family, where her mother supported her father's naval career and stayed home with Cindy and her five siblings. Many of her siblings are also in the armed services. She earned a bachelor's of science in English from the Naval Academy and holds a master's degree in mass communication and media studies (she started the latter program, which was accelerated, when her second child was one month old). Cindy is Caucasian and has two children, ages twelve and ten (eighteen months apart). She says that she is "technically" married, but she and her husband have not lived in the same state for four years. This interview was two hours in length.

APPENDIX C 173

- KRISTEN • APRIL 15, 2016 • TENNESSEE • PHONE • NAVY

A Caucasian thirty-eight-year-old, Kristen is a lieutenant commander (O-4) serving as the director of communications at Navy Personnel Command, and her husband is also in the Navy serving as an explosive ordnance disposal (EOD) technician. After three miscarriages and multiple failed intrauterine insemination (IUI) treatments, Kristen and her husband concluded she wasn't able to carry babies to term. Therefore, her pregnancy was a surprise, shortly after moving to her new assignment in Guam. Kristen's daughter is now six years old. Kristen has served for fifteen years and is very dedicated to her career, although she did express that her daughter and husband are her top priorities. Kristen loves to keep busy, evidenced by the fact that was scheduled to defend her master's thesis—examining the communication of millennial sailors—a few weeks after our interview.

- ELSA • APRIL 26, 2016 • CALIFORNIA • PHONE • NAVY

Elsa is a Caucasian thirty-three-year-old lieutenant (O-3). She has served as an aviator for almost ten and a half years and is married to a Navy aviator. Her father was also in the Navy. Elsa has two boys, ages three and a half years and two and a half months, and both were planned. Her first son was born with serious health issues, which impacted the planning of her second pregnancy. She was scheduled to graduate in the summer of 2016 with her MBA. Elsa is well informed, realistic, and dedicated. She has plans to transition out of active duty the next year or so and move to the Reserves, where she can continue flying while working in the civilian sector. She and her husband would like to have one more child.

- CLAUDIA • APRIL 27, 2016 • VIRGINIA • PHONE • NAVY
- ENLISTED & OFFICER

Claudia enlisted as a sailor, and after six years, as an E-6, went through the officer commissioning program to become an officer. She is now a lieutenant (O-3) intelligence officer and has been on active duty for a total of fourteen years. Claudia is married and has four children—the oldest are eight and four years old, and the youngest are twenty-three-month-old twins. All her pregnancies were "absolutely planned," with her first pregnancy taking place during her officer commissioning program. Claudia is a friendly thirty-five-year-old Caucasian with a bachelor's degree in global studies.

- MAE • MAY 4, 2016 • VIRGINIA • SKYPE • NAVY

Mae is an intelligence officer, and her rank is lieutenant (O-3). She is Caucasian, thirty-two years old, with a master's degree in American history and public history. She has served for five and a half years and, although she has enjoyed her time in the Navy, is planning to leave when her current order is up (in about a year) citing the difficulty of deploying as a parent as well as the incompatibility of her husband's career with the military lifestyle of constant moves. Mae is well informed and realistic in her assessment of the Navy's accommodations to pregnant and parenting servicemembers.

- TANYA • MAY 16, 2016 • VIRGINIA • SKYPE • NAVY

Tanya is Caucasian and has served seventeen and a half years as a surface warfare officer. She is a commander (O-5) in a dual-military marriage to a husband who is about to promote to commander, as well. At thirty-nine years old, she has an MA in management and human resources and has two children, a five-year-old daughter and a three-year-old son. Both of her pregnancies were (hyper)planned while she was a lieutenant commander. Tanya often serves as a mentor to servicewomen who are pregnant and/or thinking about becoming pregnant, and is very realistic about the demands and guilt that come from work-life balance. She is very career driven and deeply values being able to appreciate being pregnant, what she referred to as "one of the most joyous occasions in your personal life."

- SADIE • MAY 24, 2016 • NEW MEXICO • SKYPE • NAVY

Sadie graduated from the Naval Academy with a degree in political science. She met her husband, who is on active duty in the Air Force, while on a semester exchange program with the Air Force Academy. Sadie is thirty-three years old, Caucasian, and served eight years as an officer after graduation before becoming a Navy reservist. When she was on active duty, she worked in aviation as a helicopter pilot. She was a lieutenant (O-3) when she left active duty and has since been promoted to lieutenant commander (O-4) as a reservist. Sadie and her husband have two children, ages five and three. Her first child was born while she was on active duty and her second while she was a reservist. Sadie is very friendly and open, laughs easily, and has a clear understanding of her goals as a servicewoman and how they relate to her personal family goals.

- CANDEE • JUNE 8, 2016 • VIRGINIA • PHONE • NAVY

After graduating from the Naval Academy, Candee started her career as a surface warfare officer and later transitioned to a public affairs officer. She served twenty-five years, including her time at the Naval Academy, before retiring as a commander (O-5). Candee is forty-two years old, Caucasian, and has three children, ages seventeen, fourteen, and twelve. All her pregnancies were planned, and her first two pregnancies were when she was an active-duty lieutenant, her third while she was a lieutenant commander reservist. Candee is in a dual-military marriage, and her husband was on active duty after she transitioned to reservist. During her time in the military, Candee saw significant changes in policies that affect women, and her last assignment as active duty was at the Chief of Navy Personnel working on women's issues such as women's policies, retention of women, and women's talent management.

- PAIGE • JUNE 10, 2016 • VIRGINIA • FACETIME & PHONE • NAVY

Paige is a retired public affairs officer. Now fifty-one years old, she retired as a captain (O-6) at forty-eight years old after serving twenty-six years. The interview began on FaceTime, but because of a poor connection, we switched to the phone. Paige is Caucasian, married, and has four kids (ages twenty-three, twenty, fourteen, and ten). Her first two children are boys and her second two are girls. Both the first and last pregnancy were unplanned. For the first two pregnancies, Paige was a lieutenant (O-3), the third she was a lieutenant commander (O-4), and the fourth she was a commander (O-5). Paige is a friendly, talkative woman who laughs easily. She has two master's degrees, one from American University in broadcast journalism and one from the Naval War College in national security affairs; she was pregnant during both master's programs. Because of the age range of her children, Paige experienced many changes in Navy policies and culture, especially as it related to breastfeeding.

- FRIDA • JUNE 14, 2016 • CALIFORNIA • FACETIME • NAVY

Frida is personable, talkative, and driven. She served for twenty years before recently retiring. She was a public affairs officer and retired as a commander (O-5). We talked the week following her retirement ceremony.

When she married her husband, they were both in the Navy, but he left after eleven years so that he could provide stability at home while she pursued her military career, which she loved. Frida is forty-two, Caucasian, and has four children—ten-year-old twins (boy and girl), an eight-year-old boy, and a six-year-old boy. All her pregnancies were planned.

- GETOYA • JULY 13, 2016 • CALIFORNIA • SKYPE • NAVY
- ENLISTED & OFFICER

After enlisting in 1996, Getoya commissioned as a surface warfare officer (SWO) in 2002, and now works as a nuclear engineer. Getoya is a kind and tactful thirty-eight-year-old, Caucasian, married, and has her master's degree in international security and strategic studies. She has a ten-month-old girl at home, and was part of the small group of Navy servicewomen who received eighteen weeks of maternity leave. In addition to the support she receives from her husband and each of their families, her faith and church community are also a significant part of her life. Getoya's husband was in the background during the interview and made humorous comments. Getoya is very committed to her job, and she hopes that the Navy will soon find a way to retain more women in higher-ranking leadership positions.

- ALEXA • JULY 20, 2016 • NEW MEXICO • FACETIME
- AIR FORCE

Alexa attended the Air Force Academy before becoming an aircraft maintenance officer, a career path that has a lower percentage of women than most of the Air Force and the military. She is a captain (O-3), and has served five years since graduating from the Air Force Academy. Alexa is twenty-eight years old, Hispanic, married, and has a twenty-month-old daughter. She also informed me during the interview that she had recently discovered she was pregnant with her second child and had not told anyone yet. Alexa's first pregnancy was unplanned (she'd had an IUD to prevent pregnancy at the time while she was serving in Italy), and her second pregnancy was planned. She is very excited to be expecting a baby while she lives closer to family. In addition to her bachelor's degree, she holds an MBA in human resources management.

- **LYNN • AUGUST 19, 2016 • VIRGINIA • PHONE • AIR FORCE**

A captain (O-3) on an Aircraft Maintenance Unit, Lynn has been on active duty for five years. She attended preparatory school and the Air Force Academy (BS in management) and comes from a family that is a "long line of military," including both of her parents who served in the Air Force. Lynn is twenty-eight years old, married, and self-identifies as Black, White, and Native American. She and her husband were both military, until they were supposed to be stationed separately, so her husband chose to leave the military. Lynn and her husband have a five-month-old daughter, and she also has an eight-year-old stepdaughter. Lynn's pregnancy was unplanned. She and her husband would like to have four children, so she is trying to see if her deployment and promotion schedule will coordinate in a way that makes it possible to have four children with a successful and fulfilling military career. When we talked, Lynn was on training away from home.

- **CLEMENTINE • AUGUST 24, 2016 • GEORGIA • FACETIME**
- **AIR FORCE**

Clementine is currently a civilian, on sabbatical in the Career Intermission Program (CIP). Before separating, she had served seven years and nine months as a helicopter pilot, and was a captain (O-3). Her husband is also an Air Force pilot, and the two of them met in the Air Force Academy. Clementine is thirty years old, Caucasian, and has her master's in political science/international security (which she earned in Paris on an Air Force scholarship). Her daughter is eleven months old, and she is also five and a half months pregnant. Her first pregnancy was unplanned, but her second pregnancy was planned to coincide with CIP so that she could use the pause in her career to have her children and be with them for a couple of years before resuming her military career. When she returns, Clementine will owe the military ten more years of service (due to pilot training and CIP), which coincides with her original career goal to serve twenty years.

- **ROXANNE • FEBRUARY 14, 2017 • FLORIDA • PHONE • NAVY**

Roxanne is a pilot with a seven-month-old daughter. She is Caucasian, and, at thirty-four years old, she has served twelve and a half years and is a lieutenant commander (O-4). She has her bachelor's degree in civil engineering. Roxanne is married and also has a stepson. Unique from the other participants, Roxanne used IVF to conceive her daughter, a medical process not covered by the military's medical insurance. She is a self-proclaimed "hard-headed" person who fights for what she believes are her rights as a woman and as a service member. One of the biggest things she fought for was the right to be able to continue to fly while pregnant so that she could continue to accrue flight hours and work toward her promotion, which she received while pregnant.

Notes

CHAPTER 1. THE PREGNANCY CONTINUUM
IN THE MILITARY

1. After the issue was published, *Time* was accused of using sensationalism to boost waning readership. See Karrin Anderson, "Breast of Times, Worst of Times: 'Nursing in Uniform' Photos Draw Fire," Reading the Pictures, May 31, 2012, https://www.readingthepictures.org/2012/05/breast-of-times-worst-of-times-nursing-in-uniform-photos-draw-fire/.

2. Lylah Alphonse, "Military Moms Breastfeeding in Uniform Stir Controversy," Yahoo! Shine, May 12, 2012, http://shine.yahoo.com/parenting/military-moms-breastfeeding-uniform-stir-controversey-214500503.html.

3. Joanna Walters, "Yahoo CEO Marissa Mayer's Minimal Maternity Leave Plan Prompts Dismay," *The Guardian*, September 3, 2015, sec. Technology, http://www.theguardian.com/technology/2015/sep/02/yahoo-ceo-marissa-mayer-minimal-maternity-leave-plan-prompts-dismay.

4. Jennifer Borda, "Lean in or Leave before You Leave?: False Dichotomies of Choice and Blame in Public Debates about Working Motherhood," in *The Mother Blame-Game*, ed. Vanessa Reimer and Sahagian (Toronto, ON: Demeter Press, 2005), 219–36; Sheryl Sandberg and Nell Scovall,

Lean In: Women, Work, and the Will to Lead (New York: Alfred A. Knopf, 2013).

5. Patrice M. Buzzanell et al., "The Good *Working* Mother: Managerial Women's Sensemaking and Feelings about Work-Family Issues," *Communication Studies* 56, no. 3 (January 2005): 261-85, https://doi.org/10.1080/10510970500181389.

6. Joan Acker, "Hierarchies, Jobs, Bodies: A Theory of Gendered Organizations," *Gender & Society* 4, no. 2 (June 1, 1990): 139-58, https://doi.org/10.1177/089124390004002002. Acker discusses how organizational structures—and specifically hierarchical organizations—cannot be assumed to be gender neutral; rather, gendered assumptions underlie organizational structures and policies, wherein the disembodied/neutral worker is always already male. Therefore, to function at the top of an organizational hierarchy, one must display hegemonic masculinity, which "requires that women render irrelevant everything that makes them women" (153). These larger patriarchal foundations of gender and power in organizations—and their impact on women and women's bodies particularly—will be discussed in more depth throughout this book.

7. Although the military has changed its language regarding personnel from "servicewomen" and "servicemen" to "female service member" and "male service member," I use the colloquial verbiage of "servicewoman."

8. Megan D. McFarlane, "Breastfeeding as Subversive: Mothers, Mammaries, and the Military," *International Feminist Journal of Politics*, January 29, 2014, 1-18.

9. Elizabeth C. Britt, *Conceiving Normalcy: Rhetoric, Law, and the Double Binds of Infertility*, (Tuscaloosa: University of Alabama Press, 2001); Koerber, *Breast or Bottle?: Contemporary Controversies in Infant-Feeding Policy and Practice* (Columbia: University of South Carolina Press, 2013); Sarah Projansky, *Spectacular Girls: Media Fascination and Celebrity Culture* (New York: New York University Press, 2014); Elizabeth C. Britt, *Reimagining Advocacy: Rhetorical Education in the Legal Clinic* (University Park: Penn State University Press, 2018).

10. Raymie E. McKerrow, "Critical Rhetoric: Theory and Praxis," *Communication Monographs* 56 (June 1989): 91-111; Michael Calvin McGee, "Text, Context, and the Fragmentation of Contemporary Culture," *Western Journal of Speech Communication* 54, Summer (1990): 274-89.

11. Maurice Charland, "Constitutive Rhetoric: The Case of the Peuple Québécois," *Quarterly Journal of Speech* 73, no. 2 (1987): 133-50; McGee, "Text, Context, and the Fragmentation of Contemporary Culture."

12. Britt, *Reimagining Advocacy*, 3.

13. McKerrow, "Critical Rhetoric."

14. Sonja K. Foss, *Rhetorical Criticism: Exploration and Practice*, 5th ed. (Long Grove, IL: Waveland Press, 2017); James Jasinski, *Sourcebook on Rhetoric: Key Concepts in Contemporary Rhetorical Studies* (Thousand Oaks, CA: SAGE, 2001); Jack Selzer, "Rhetorical Analysis: Understanding How Texts Persuade Readers," in *What Writing Does and How It Does It*, ed. Charles Bazerman and Paul Prior (Mahwah, NJ: Lawrence Erlbaum, 2004), 279–30.

15. Cynthia Enloe, *Globalization and Militarism: Feminists Make the Link* (Lanham, MD: Rowman & Littlefield, 2007).

16. Allison Yarrow, "Shaheen Amendment Expands Female Service Members' Access to Abortion," *The Daily Beast*, January 3, 2013, http://www.thedailybeast.com/articles/2013/01/03/shaheen-amendment-expands-female-service-members-access-to-abortion.html.

17. It should be noted that this approach differs from critical rhetoric analyses of marginalized rhetorical communities, such as the work of Kent Ono and John M. Sloop ("The Critique of Vernacular Discourse," *Communication Monographs* 62, no. 1 [1995]: 19–46) because I conducted and analyzed personal interviews with some who are in the marginalized rhetorical community. It also differs from the work of many rhetorical ethnographers and those employing participatory critical rhetoric because it does not include interactions in situ, but rather retrospective interviews conducted in-person, as well as mediated by technology such as telephones, Skype, and FaceTime. See, e.g., Michael Middleton et al., *Participatory Critical Rhetoric: Theoretical and Methodological Foundations for Studying Rhetoric In Situ* (Lanham, MD: Lexington, 2017); Michael Middleton, Samantha Senda-Cook, and Danielle Endres, "Articulating Rhetorical Field Methods: Challenges and Tensions," *Western Journal of Communication* 75, no. 4 (July 2011): 386–406.

18. Donna Haraway, "Situated Knowledges: The Science Question in Feminism and the Privilege of Partial Perspectives," *Feminist Studies* 14, no. 3 (1988): 575–99.

19. Sharlene Hesse-Biber, "A Re-Invitation of Feminist Research," in *Feminist Research Practice: A Primer*, ed. Sharlene Hesse-Biber, 2nd. ed. (Los Angeles: SAGE, 2014), 1–13. To be clear, this method does not allow for the achievement of discovering "the truth" about servicewomen's experiences, but rather shows the multiplicity of experiences and how they are similar, different, and overlap. In my analysis, themes did emerge from the

interviews with servicewomen regarding their pregnancy experiences, and there were also contradictions between servicewomen's experiences.

20. Snowball sampling is a qualitative interviewing method wherein researchers identify several participants "who fit the study's criteria and then ask these people to suggest a colleague, a friend, or a family member." See Sarah J. Tracy, *Qualitative Research Methods: Collecting Evidence, Crafting Analysis, Communicating Impact* (Malden: Wiley-Blackwell, 2013).

21. To read more about the interviewees' demographics, as well as the profiles of interviewees, please see the appendixes.

22. Patrice M. Buzzanell and Laura L. Ellingson, "Contesting Narratives of Workplace Maternity," in *Narratives, Health, and Healing: Communication Theory, Research, and Practice*, ed. Lynn M Harter, Phyllis M. Japp, and Christina S. Beck (Mahwah, NJ: Lawrence Earlbaum, 2004), 277–94; Patrice M. Buzzanell and Meina Liu, "It's 'Give and Take': Maternity Leave as a Conflict Management Process," *Human Relations* 60, no. 3 (March 1, 2007): 465, https://doi.org/10.1177/0018726707076688; Patrice M. Buzzanell and Meina Liu, "Struggling with Maternity Leave Policies and Practices: A Poststructuralist Feminist Analysis of Gendered Organizing," *Journal of Applied Communication Research* 33, no. 1 (February 2005): 1–25, https://doi.org/10.1080/0090988042000318495; Buzzanell et al., "The Good *Working* Mother"; Karen Lee Ashcraft, "Managing Maternity Leave: A Qualitative Analysis of Temporary Executive Succession," *Administrative Science Quarterly* 44 (1999): 240–80.

23. George Cheney and Daniel J. Lair, "Theorizing about Rhetoric and Organizations," in *Engaging Organizational Communication Theory and Research: Multiple Perspectives*, ed. Steve May and Dennis K. Mumby (Thousand Oaks, CA: SAGE, 2005), 55–84, http://dx.doi.org/10.4135/9781452204536.n4.

24. Susan A. Owen and Peter Ehrenhaus, "Animating a Critical Rhetoric: On the Feeding Habits of American Empire," *Western Journal of Communication* 57, no. Spring (1993): 169–77; Dilip Parameshwar Gaonkar, "Performing with Fragments: Reflections on Critical Rhetoric," *Argument and the Postmodern Challenge: Proceedings from the Eighth SCA/AFA Conference on Argumentation*, 1993, 149–55; Kevin Michael DeLuca, *Image Politics the New Rhetoric of Environmental Activism* (Mahwah, NJ: Lawrence Erlbaum, 1999); Phaedra C. Pezzullo, "Performing Critical Interruptions: Stories, Rhetorical Invention, and the Environmental Justice Movement," *Western Journal of Communication* 65, no. 1 (March 2001): 1–25, https://doi.org/10.1080/10570310109374689.

25. The focus of this book is on the embodied pregnancy experience of women in the U.S. military, yet I acknowledge that biological reproduction is not the only path to motherhood/parenting, and much research can be done on adoption planning and foster/guardianship within the military.

26. Guenter-Schlesinger, "Persistence of Sexual Harassment: The Impact of Military Culture on Policy Implementation," in *Beyond Zero Tolerance: Discrimination in Military Culture*, ed. Mary Fainsod Katzenstein and Judith Reppy (Lanham, MD: Rowman & Littlefield, 1999), 195.

27. Stephen Losey, "New Air Force Policy Gives New Mothers 12 Months to Decide If They Want to Stay in Uniform," *Air Force Times*, April 29, 2017, https://www.airforcetimes.com/news/your-air-force/2017/04/29/new-air-force-policy-gives-new-mothers-12-months-to-decide-if-they-want-to-stay-in-uniform/; Kristy N. Kamarck, "Women in Combat: Issues for Congress," Congressional Research Service, December 3, 2015, https://fas.org/sgp/crs/natsec/R42075.pdf; Courtney Kube and Jim Miklaszewski, "Military to Announce Changes to Maternity Leave Policy," NBC News, January 28, 2016, http://www.nbcnews.com/news/us-news/military-announce-changes-maternity-leave-policy-n506006; Amy Bushatz, "Breastfeeding Policy Will Help Army Retain Female Soldiers: Lawmaker," Military.Com, December 17, 2015, http://www.military.com/daily-news/2015/12/17/breastfeeding-policy-help-army-retain-female-soldiers-lawmaker.html; Andrew Tilghman and David Larter, "New 12-Week Maternity Policy for All Services Means Big Cut for Navy, Marines," *Navy Times*, January 28, 2016, http://www.navytimes.com/story/military/2016/01/28/maternity-leave-dod-ash-carter-12-weeks-announcement-force-of-the-future/79465178/.

28. Brian Wagner, "The Military Could Soon Face Increased Recruiting Challenges," *Task and Purpose*, February 18, 2016, https://taskandpurpose.com/the-military-could-soon-face-increased-recruiting-challenges/; Tom Vanden Brook, "Army to Spend $300 Million on Bonuses and Ads to Get 6,000 More Recruits," *USA Today*, February 12, 2017, https://www.usatoday.com/story/news/politics/2017/02/12/army-spend-300-million-bonuses-and-ads-get-6000-more-recruits/97757094/; Fred Kaplan, "The U.S. Army Lowers Recruitment Standards . . . Again," *Slate*, January 24, 2008, http://www.slate.com/articles/news_and_politics/war_stories/2008/01/dumb_and_dumber.html.

29. Natalie Kitroeff, "Why Are So Many Women Dropping Out of the Workforce?," *Los Angeles Times*, May 28, 2017, http://www.latimes.com/business/la-fi-women-dropping-out-20170522-story.html; Alex

Mahadevan, "Women Are Leaving the Workforce at a Staggering Rate—Here's Why," *The Penny Hoarder*, August 23, 2017, http://www.thepennyhoarder.com/make-money/shrinking-number-of-women-in-the-workforce/.

30. R. Lee Biggs et al., "The Impact of Pregnancy on the Individual and Military Organization: A Postpartum Active Duty Survey," *Military Medicine* 174, no. 1 (2009): 64.

31. "The Military Is Pregnant: Coping with Motherhood in the Armed Forces," *Time*, October 8, 1979.

32. Jennifer Hickes Lundquist and Herbert L. Smith, "Family Formation among Women in the US Military: Evidence from the NLSY," *Journal of Marriage and Family* 67, no. 1 (2005): 2.

33. April S. Fitzgerald et al., "A Primer on the Unique Challenges of Female Soldiers' Reproductive Issues in a War-Ready Culture," *Military Medicine* 178, no. 5 (May 2013): 511–16, https://doi.org/10.7205/MILMED-D-12-00384.

34. This is made even more problematic given the high rates of rape and sexual assault in the military, which can result in pregnancy.

35. Laurie A. Kwolek, Cristobal S. Berry-Caban, and Sean F. Thomas, "Pregnant Soldiers' Participation in Physical Training: A Descriptive Study," *Military Medicine* 176, no. 8 (2011): 926–31.

36. Kelsey Holt et al., "Unintended Pregnancy and Contraceptive Use among Women in the US Military: A Systematic Literature Review," *Military Medicine* 176, no. 9 (2011): 1056.

37. See, e.g., Buzzanell et al., "The Good *Working* Mother"; D. Lynn O'Brien Hallstein, "Silences and Choice: The Legacies of White Second Wave Feminism in the New Professoriate," *Women's Studies in Communication* 31, no. 2 (July 2008): 143–50, https://doi.org/10.1080/07491409.2008.10162526; D. Lynn O'Brien Hallstein, "Introduction to Mothering Rhetorics," *Women's Studies in Communication* 40, no. 1 (2017): 1–10, http://dx.doi.org/10.1080/07491409.2017.1280326; D. Lynn O'Brien Hallstein, "Public Choices, Private Control: How Mediated Mom Labels Work Rhetorically to Dismantle the Politics of Choice and White Second Wave Feminist Successes," in *Contemplating Maternity in an Era of Choice: Explorations into Discourses of Reproduction*, ed. Sara Hayden and D. Lynn O'Brien Hallstein (Lanham, MD: Lexington Books, 2010), 5–26; Sharon Hays, *The Cultural Contradictions of Motherhood* (New Haven, CT: Yale University Press, 1996); Susan Douglas and Meredith Michaels, *The Mommy Myth: The Idealization of Motherhood and How*

It Has Undermined All Women (New York: Free Press, 2004); Ashley N. Mack, "Disciplining Mommy: Rhetorics of Reproduction in Contemporary Maternity Culture," PhD diss., University of Texas at Austin, 2013, http://repositories.lib.utexas.edu/bitstream/ handle/2152/21299/MACK-DISSERTATION-2013.pdf?sequence=1; Lindal Buchanan, *Rhetorics of Motherhood* (Carbondale: Southern Illinois University Press, 2013); Diane Eyer, *Motherguilt: How Our Culture Blames Mothers for What's Wrong with Society* (New York: Random House, 1996).

38. William Tangney, "Recruitment, Retention, & Readiness," *Army Magazine* 49, no. 3 (March 1999): 15.

39. Michael R. Duke and Genevieve M. Ames, "Challenges of Contraceptive Use and Pregnancy Prevention among Women in the U.S. Navy," *Qualitative Health Research* 18, no. 2 (February 1, 2008): 244–53, https://doi.org/10.1177/1049732307312305.

40. Buzzanell and Liu, "It's 'Give and Take.'"

41. Buzzanell and Ellingson, "Contesting Narratives of Workplace Maternity," 277.

42. Biggs et al., "The Impact of Pregnancy," 64.

43. Taber, "'You Better Not Get Pregnant While You're Here': Tensions between Masculinities and Femininities in Military Communities of Practice," *International Journal of Lifelong Education* 30, no. 3 (June 2011): 331–48, https://doi.org/10.1080/02601370.2011.570871; Ginny Carroll and Carol Barkalow, "Women Have What It Takes," *Newsweek*, August 5, 1991; Joshua S. Goldstein, *War and Gender: How Gender Shapes the War System and Vice Versa* (Cambridge: Cambridge University Press, 2001); Penny F. Pierce, "The Role of Women in the Military," in *Military Life: Military Culture*, ed. Thomas W. Britt, Amy B. Adler, and Carl Andrew Castro (Westport, CT: Greenwood Publishing Group, 2006), 97–118.

44. Patricia J. Thomas and Marie D. Thomas, "Effects of Sex, Marital Status, and Parental Status on Absenteeism among Navy Enlisted Personnel," *Military Psychology* 6, no. 2 (1994): 95.

45. Carol Burke, "Military Folk Culture," in Katzenstein and Reppy, *Beyond Zero Tolerance*, 53–63; Karen O. Dunivan, "Military Culture: Change and Continuity," *Armed Forces & Society* 20, no. 4 (1994): 531–47; Guenter-Schlesinger, "Persistence of Sexual Harassment"; Madeline Morris, "In War and Peace: Incidence and Implications of Rape by Military Personnel," in Katzenstein and Reppy, *Beyond Zero Tolerance*, 163–94; Paul E. Roush, "A Tangled Webb the Navy Can't Afford," in Katzenstein and Reppy, *Beyond Zero Tolerance*, 81–99.

46. Melissa T. Brown, *Enlisting Masculinity: The Construction of Gender in US Military Recruiting Advertising during the All-Volunteer Force* (New York: Oxford University Press, 2012).

47. Michael S. Kimmel, "Masculinity as Homophobia," in *The Social Construction of Difference and Inequality*, ed. T. E. Ore, 2nd ed. (Boston: McGraw-Hill, 2003), 119–36.

48. Brown, *Enlisting Masculinity*, 19.

49. Goldstein, *War and Gender*.

50. Frank J. Barrett, "The Organizational Construction of Hegemonic Masculinity: The Case of the US Navy," *Gender, Work & Organization* 3, no. 3 (1996): 129–42; Brown, *Enlisting Masculinity*; R. W. Connell, *Masculinities*, 2nd ed. (Berkeley: University of California Press, 2005); R. W. Connell, "Masculinity, Violence, and War," in *War/Masculinity*, ed. Paul Patton and Ross Poole (Sydney, Australia: Intervention, 1985); Joe Dubbert, *Man's Place: Masculinity in Transition* (Englewood Cliffs, NJ: Prentice Hall, 1979); Cynthia Enloe, "Beyond Steve Canyon and Rambo: Feminist Histories of Militarized Masculinity," in *Militarization of the Western World*, ed. John Gillis (New Brunswick, NJ: Rutgers University Press, 1989), 119–40; Paul Higate, *Military Masculinities: Identity and the State* (Westport, CT: Praeger, 2003); Christina S. Jarvis, *The Male Body at War: American Masculinity during World War II* (DeKalb: Northern Illinois University Press, 2010); Mary Fainsod Katzenstein and Judith Reppy, eds., *Beyond Zero Tolerance: Discrimination in Military Culture* (Lanham, MD: Rowman & Littlefield, 1999; David H. Morgan, "Theater of War: Combat, the Military, and Masculinities," in *Theorizing Masculinities*, ed. Harry Brod and Michael Kaufman (Thousand Oaks, CA: SAGE, 1994, 165–82; Sandra Whitworth, "Militarized Masculinity and Post-Traumatic Stress Disorder," in *Rethinking the Man Question: Sex, Gender and Violence in International Relations*, ed. Jane L. Parpart and Marysia Zalewski (London: Zed Books, 2008), 109–26.

51. Carole Pateman, "The Fraternal Social Contract," in *The Disorder of Women: Democracy, Feminism, and Political Theory* (Stanford, CA: Stanford University Press, 1990), 49.

52. Brown, *Enlisting Masculinity*.

53. Enloe, *Globalization and Militarism*, 71.

54. Paula A. Johnson, Sheila E. Widnall, and Frazier F. Benya, eds., *Sexual Harassment of Women: Climate, Culture, and Consequences in Academic Sciences, Engineering, and Medicine* (Washington, DC: The National Academies Press, 2018).

55. Elizabeth Comack and Tracey Peter, "How the Criminal Justice System Responds to Sexual Assault Survivors: The Slippage between 'Responsibilization' and 'Blaming the Victim,'" *Canadian Journal of Women and the Law* 17, no. 2 (2005): 283–309, https://doi.org/10.1353/jwl.2007.0002.

56. Kelly Hannah-Moffat, *Punishment in Disguise: Penal Governance and Federal Imprisonment of Women in Canada* (Toronto: University of Toronto Press, 2001), 172.

57. G. C. Gray, "The Responsibilization Strategy of Health and Safety: Neo-Liberalism and the Reconfiguration of Individual Responsibility for Risk," *British Journal of Criminology* 49, no. 3 (January 6, 2009): 329, https://doi.org/10.1093/bjc/azp004.

58. Natalie Fixmer-Oraiz, "Contemplating Homeland Maternity," *Women's Studies in Communication* 38, no. 2 (April 3, 2015): 129–34.

59. Comack and Peter, "How the Criminal Justice System Responds"; Gray, "The Responsibilization Strategy."

60. Sara Hayden and D. Lynn O'Brien Hallstein, "Introduction," in *Contemplating Maternity in an Era of Choice: Explorations into Discourses of Reproduction*, ed. Sara Hayden and D. Lynn O'Brien Hallstein (Lanham, MD: Lexington Books, 2010), xviii.

61. Natalie Fixmer-Oraiz, *Homeland Maternity: US Security Culture and the New Reproductive Regime* (Urbana: University of Illinois Press, 2019).

62. Russel Read, "Why the US Military Is on the Brink of a Recruitment Crisis," WJLA, February 16, 2018, http://wjla.com/news/nation-world/why-the-us-military-is-on-the-brink-of-a-recruitment-crisis.

63. Fixmer-Oraiz, "Contemplating Homeland Maternity," 15.

64. Fixmer-Oraiz, *Homeland Maternity*, 14.

65. Michel Foucault, *Discipline and Punish: The Birth of the Prison*, 2nd ed. (New York: Vintage, 1995), 136.

66. John Blake Scott, *Risky Rhetoric: AIDS and the Cultural Practices of HIV Testing* (Carbondale: Southern Illinois University Press, 2003), 7–8.

67. Fixmer-Oraiz, *Homeland Maternity*, 23.

68. Mack, "Disciplining Mommy," 4.

69. Mack, "Disciplining Mommy," 4.

70. Mack, "Disciplining Mommy"; Sharon Hays, *The Cultural Contradictions of Motherhood* (New Haven, CT: Yale University Press, 1996); Diane Eyer, *Motherguilt*.

71. Several books in recent decades have examined rhetorics of mothering/motherhood. These include Hays's groundbreaking book,

which discusses the cultural contradictions of mothering, specifically referring to the cultural contradiction between home and work. See Hays, *The Cultural Contradictions of Motherhood*. Douglas and Michaels' examination of what they call "the new momism," or the increasing intensity associated with motherhood that has gained speed in media representations since the 1980s, is also a foundational text on the analysis of cultural constructions of motherhood through the media. See Douglas and Michaels, *The Mommy Myth*. Eyer's book argues that much of society's problems—including welfare, child poverty, riots, divorce—are blamed on mothers. See Eyer, *Motherguilt*. Recently, in the field of communication studies specifically, Hayden and O'Brien Hallstein's edited volume contains essays from communication scholars who examine modern-day maternity in light of the "era of choice" at the end of the twentieth century and Buchanan uses a feminist rhetorical lens to examine the topic of motherhood. See Sara Hayden and D. Lynn O'Brien Hallstein, eds., *Contemplating Maternity in an Era of Choice: Explorations into Discourses of Reproduction* (Lanham, MD: Lexington Books, 2010); Buchanan, *Rhetorics of Motherhood*. All of these books informed this project. My approach to studying maternity differs from these books in that I utilize a multimethod approach that combines interviews with rhetorical analysis to look specifically at women in the military, as opposed to women's work/life balance in general.

72. Foucault, *Discipline and Punish*, 23, 183.

73. Nollaig Frost and Frauke Elichaoff, "Feminist Postmodernism, Poststructuralism, and Critical Theory," in *Feminist Research Practice: A Primer*, ed. Sharlene Hesse-Biber (Los Angeles, CA: SAGE Publications, 2014).

74. Mack, "Disciplining Mommy," 17.

75. Biggs et al., "The Impact of Pregnancy on the Individual," 64.

76. Guenter-Schlesinger, "Persistence of Sexual Harassment," 195.

77. Enloe, *Globalization and Militarism*.

78. Katzenstein and Reppy, *Beyond Zero Tolerance*.

79. Johnson, Widnall, and Benya, *Sexual Harassment of Women*.

80. Johnson, Widnall, and Benya, *Sexual Harassment of Women*, 123.

81. Megan D. McFarlane, "Circuits of Discipline: Intensified Responsibilization and the Double Bind of Pregnancy in the U.S. Military," *Women's Studies in Communication* 41, no. 1 (January 2, 2018): 22–41, https://doi.org/10.1080/07491409.2017.1419525; In some ways, my argument and use of "circuit" resonates with Haraway's discussion of how women are

constituted within the "integrated circuit." Whereas Haraway is more concerned with the way science and technology restructure the social relations of women and many social locations (like the home, market, school, clinic-hospital, etc.), I explore specifically how a loop of discipline is created within the military workplace that produces "responsible pregnant (service)women" who in turn reify this double-bind of responsibilization. Donna Haraway, *Simians, Cyborgs, and Women: The Reinvention of Nature* (New York: Routledge, 1991).

82. Previous studies on women's relationships with the military have examined how the military affects civilian women and servicewomen, with one of the leaders in these studies being Cynthia Enloe. Much of her research has more of a global focus on Western military forces and the effects of masculinity in the military. See, e.g., Enloe, *Globalization and Militarism*; Enloe, "Beyond Steve Canyon and Rambo"; Enloe, *Maneuvers: The International Politics of Militarizing Women's Lives* (Berkeley, CA: University of California Press, 2000); Enloe, *Does Khaki Become You?: The Militarisation of Women's Lives* (London: Pluto Press Limited, 1983); See also Taber, "'You Better Not Get Pregnant While You're Here.'"

Other studies have focused on U.S. servicewomen. For example, retired Major General Jeanne Holm focused on the history and role of servicewomen in *Women in the Military: An Unfinished Revolution* (New York: Presidio Press, 1993). In her book, Holm walks readers through the history of women in the military since the Revolutionary War, showing how women's roles have developed and changed. In a more recent book, *Undaunted: The Real Story of America's Servicewomen in Today's Military* (New York: Penguin, 2014), Tanya Biank, a journalist and wife, sister, and daughter of military servicemembers, takes a journalistic and narrative approach to tell the stories of four active-duty servicewomen. Her in-depth storytelling of these women's lives over the course of a few years in each of their careers attempts to move past stereotypes and caricatures and show the choices, contradictions, and difficulties of being a woman in the paradoxical culture of the military, which is a "curious mix of traditional men and unconventional women" (p. 5). Although one servicewoman's story includes the difficulty of leaving children behind and trying to manage a struggling marriage in a dual-military career family, the book focuses much more on each woman's story, showing the different paths that lead women to join the armed forces, and the different experiences therein. A more maternal focus is given in a book by U.S. Navy veteran, Robyn Roche-Paull, *Breastfeeding in Combat Boots: A Survival Guide to Successful Breastfeeding while Serving in the US Military* (CreateSpace Independent Publish Platform). This book is written by and for women in the military who are pregnant and either contemplating breastfeeding or trying to understand their options and rights when it comes to breastfeeding in the military.

83. Biggs et al., "The Impact of Pregnancy on the Individual"; Duke and Ames, "Challenges of Contraceptive Use"; Mary Ann Evans and Leora Rosen, "Pregnancy Planning and the Impact on Work Climate, Psychological Well-Being, and Work Effort in the Military," *Journal of Occupational Health Psychology* 2, no. 4 (1997): 353; Meg Gerrard, Frederick X. Gibbons, and Teddy D. Warner, "Effects of Reviewing Risk-Relevant Behavior on Perceived Vulnerability among Women Marines," *Health Psychology* 10, no. 3 (1991): 173; Kelsey Holt et al., "Unintended Pregnancy and Contraceptive Use among Women in the US Military: A Systematic Literature Review," *Military Medicine* 176, no. 9 (2011): 1056–64; Janet C. Jacobson and Jeffrey T. Jensen, "A Policy of Discrimination: Reproductive Health Care in the Military," *Women's Health Issues* 21, no. 4 (July 2011): 255–58, https://doi.org/10.1016/j.whi.2011.03.008; Kwolek et al., "Pregnant Soldiers' Participation in Physical Training"; Thomas and Thomas, "Effects of Sex, Marital Status, and Parental Status on Absenteeism"; Ryan J. Heitmann et al., "Unintended Pregnancy in the Military Health Care System: Who Is Really at Risk?," *Military Medicine* 181, no. 10 (October 2016): 1370–74, https://doi.org/10.7205/MILMED-D-16-00003.

84. Genevra Pittman, "Unintended Pregnancies on the Rise in Servicewomen," Reuters, January 24, 2013, http://www.reuters.com/article/2013/01/24/us-pregnancies-servicewoman-idUSBRE90N1B820130124.

85. Holt et al., "Unintended Pregnancy and Contraceptive Use"; Catherine Pearson, "Unplanned Pregnancies among Women in Military High, Rising," *Huffington Post*, January 23, 2013, sec. Women, http://www.huffingtonpost.com/2013/01/23/pregnant-military-unplanned-women_n_2534873.html; Pittman, "Unintended Pregnancies on the Rise in Servicewomen."

86. Examples of this include abortion policies, with more recent examples including paid maternity leave. See McFarlane, "U.S. Military Policy and the Discursive Construction of Servicewomen's Bodies," ProQuest Dissertations Publishing, 2015, and chapter 5 for more details.

87. Katzenstein and Reppy, *Beyond Zero Tolerance*, 3.

88. Regina Titunik, "Discrimination and Military Culture," *H-Net Reviews*, 2000, 1–3.

89. Johnson, Widnall, and Benya, *Sexual Harassment of Women*, 121.

90. Robert L. Ivie, "Productive Criticism Then and Now," *American Communication Journal* 4, no. 3 (2001), http://ac-journal.org/journal/vol4/iss3/special/ivie.pdf.
91. Fixmer-Oraiz, *Homeland Maternity*, 158.
92. Burke, "Military Folk Culture," 62.

CHAPTER 2. CONTEXTUALIZING MILITARY MATERNITY

1. *Flores vs. Secretary of Defense*, 355 Federal Supplement 93 (United States District Court for the Northern District of Florida, Pensacola Division 1973).
2. Susan Zaeske, *Signatures of Citizenship: Petitioning, Antislavery, and Women's Political Identity* (Chapel Hill: University of North Carolina Press, 2003).
3. *Flores vs. Secretary of Defense*.
4. Linda Strite Murnane, "Legal Impediments to Service: Women in the Military and the Rule of Law," *Duke Journal Gender Law & Policy* 14 (2007): 1073.
5. Joanne Martin, "Deconstructing Organizational Taboos: The Suppression of Gender Conflict in Organizations," *Organization Science* 1, no. 4 (1990), http://www.jstor.org/stable/pdf/2634968.pdf.
6. Zaeske, *Signatures of Citizenship*. It should be noted that these assumptions are racially biased. For example, whereas most White women did not work, Black women have historically been expected to work. See Nina Banks, "Black Women's Labor Market History Reveals Deep-Seated Race and Gender Discrimination," Economic Policy Institute, February 19, 2019, https://www.epi.org/blog/black-womens-labor-market-history-reveals-deep-seated-race-and-gender-discrimination/.
7. Jean Bethke Elshtain, *Women and War* (with a new epilogue) (Chicago: University of Chicago Press, 1995); Zaeske, *Signatures of Citizenship*.
8. Murnane, "Legal Impediments to Service," 1065.
9. Leslie Nemo, "The Challenge of Accessing Birth Control in the Military," *The Atlantic*, February 23, 2017, https://www.theatlantic.com/health/archive/2017/02/military-women-birth-control/517452/.
10. Stephanie Russell-Kraft, "The Double Standard of Military Pregnancy: What Contraceptive Access Won't Fix," *Rewire News*, August 2, 2016, https://rewire.news/article/2016/08/02/double-standard-military-pregnancy-what-contraceptive-access-wont-fix/; Eric Bradner, "U.S. Military Opens Combat Positions to Women," CNN.com, December 3, 2015,

https://www.cnn.com/2015/12/03/politics/u-s-military-women-combat-positions/index.html.

11. Russell-Kraft, "The Double Standard of Military Pregnancy."

12. Karen Lee Ashcraft, "Managing Maternity Leave: A Qualitative Analysis of Temporary Executive Succession," *Administrative Science Quarterly* 44 (1999): 244.

13. Murnane, "Legal Impediments to Service."

14. Cynthia Enloe, *Does Khaki Become You?: The Militarisation of Women's Lives* (London: Pluto Press Limited, 1983); Murnane, "Legal Impediments to Service."

15. Murnane, "Legal Impediments to Service."

16. This act was passed one month before Executive Order 9981 that integrated the military on the basis of race, religion, and national origin.

17. Murnane, "Legal Impediments to Service," 1067; Women's Armed Services Integration Act of 1948: Public Law No. 80-625, 62 Stat. 368, June 12, 1948, https://www.mcu.usmc.mil/historydivision/Pages/Speeches/PublicLaw625.aspx.

18. In November of 1967, President Lyndon Johnson signed into law the most significant legislative change for women in the military since WASIA, reducing some of the barriers women faced, such as lifting the legal ceiling so that women could achieve the ranks denied earlier, as well as eliminating the 2 percent cap on women's representation in the military. Yet women were still segregated into separate corps, given unequal pay, and excluded from military academies (Murnane, "Legal Impediments to Service"). Additionally, service secretaries still possessed the authority to discharge women from the service if they were pregnant, which prompted multiple court cases in the following years, such as *Flores* noted at the beginning of the chapter. April S. Fitzgerald et al., "A Primer on the Unique Challenges of Female Soldiers' Reproductive Issues in a War-Ready Culture," *Military Medicine* 178, no. 5 (May 2013): 511–16, https://doi.org/10.7205/MILMED-D-12-00384.

19. Murnane, "Legal Impediments to Service," 1067; "Women's Armed Services Integration Act of 1948," sec. 214.

20. Jeanne Holm, *Women in the Military: An Unfinished Revolution* (New York: Presidio Press, 1993), 289.

21. Harry S. Truman, "Executive Order 10240—Regulations Governing the Separation from the Service of Certain Women Serving in the Regular Army, Navy, Marine Corps, or Air Force," in *The American Presidency Project*, edited by Gerhard Peters and John T. Woolley, April 27,

1951, https://www.presidency.ucsb.edu/documents/executive-order-10240-regulations-governing-the-separation-from-the-service-certain-women.

22. Truman, "Executive Order 10240," para. 2.

23. Holm, *Women in the Military*, 292 (italics added).

24. Natalie Fixmer-Oraiz, *Homeland Maternity: US Security Culture and the New Reproductive Regime* (Urbana: University of Illinois Press, 2019).

25. Holm, *Women in the Military*, 291. Swanson also attempted to debunk misconceptions about menopause, as well. At a Senate Armed Services Committee Hearing on July 2, 1947, when it was asked if "women's incapacitation during menopause would lead to an excessive number of disability retirements," he responded that "the commonly held idea that women are invalided in their middle years by the onset of menopause is largely a popular fallacy. It is well known that men pass through the same physiological change with symptomology closely resembling that of women." See "Swanson, Dr. Clifford, RADM," https://navy.togetherweserved.com/usn/servlet/tws.webapp.WebApp?cmd=ShadowBoxProfile&type=Person&ID=510505 for more information.

26. Holm, *Women in the Military*, 291.

27. Murnane, "Legal Impediments to Service."

28. See further discussion on planned and unplanned pregnancies in chapter 3.

29. Sharon Hays, *The Cultural Contradictions of Motherhood* (New Haven, CT: Yale University Press, 1996).

30. Rebecca Todd Peters, *Trust Women: A Progressive Christian Argument for Reproductive Justice* (Boston: Beacon Press, 2018).

31. Mary Blair-Loy, "Cultural Constructions of Family Schemas: The Case of Women Finance Executives," *Gender & Society* 15, no. 5 (2001): 687.

32. *Crawford v. Cushman*, 531 Federal Reporter 1114 (United States Court of Appeals Second Circuit 1976).

33. Murnane, "Legal Impediments to Service."

34. Jennifer Hickes Lundquist and Herbert L. Smith, "Family Formation among Women in the US Military: Evidence from the NLSY." *Journal of Marriage and Family* 67, no. 1 (2005): 1–13; M. R. Duke and G. M. Ames, "Challenges of Contraceptive Use and Pregnancy Prevention among Women in the U.S. Navy," *Qualitative Health Research* 18, no. 2 (February 1, 2008): 244–53, https://doi.org/10.1177/1049732307312305.

35. R. Lee Biggs et al., "The Impact of Pregnancy on the Individual and Military Organization: A Postpartum Active Duty Survey," *Military*

Medicine 174, no. 1 (2009): 61–75; Patricia A. Thomas and Marie D. Thomas, "Effects of Sex, Marital Status, and Parental Status on Absenteeism among Navy Enlisted Personnel," *Military Psychology* 6, no. 2 (1994): 107.

36. Lundquist and Smith, "Family Formation among Women in the US Military."

37. Janet C. Jacobson and Jeffrey T. Jensen, "A Policy of Discrimination: Reproductive Health Care in the Military," *Women's Health Issues* 21, no. 4 (July 2011): 255–58, https://doi.org/10.1016/j.whi.2011.03.008; Lundquist and Smith, "Family Formation among Women in the US Military."

38. Biggs et al., "The Impact of Pregnancy on the Individual and Military Organization"; Thomas and Thomas, "Effects of Sex, Marital Status, and Parental Status," 107.

39. Mark D. Faram, "Sweeping Uniform Changes Emphasize Gender Neutrality," *Navy Times*, August 22, 2017, https://www.navytimes.com/news/your-navy/2015/10/09/sweeping-uniform-changes-emphasize-gender-neutrality/.

40. Simone de Beauvoir, *The Second Sex* (New York: Vintage, 1989); Carole Pateman, "The Fraternal Social Contract," in *The Disorder of Women: Democracy, Feminism, and Political Theory* (Stanford, CA: Stanford University Press, 1990); Elizabeth V. Spelman, "Gender & Race: The Ampersand Problem in Feminist Thought" in *Inessential Woman* (Boston: Beacon Press, 1988), 114–209.

41. Nancy Taber, "'You Better Not Get Pregnant While You're Here': Tensions between Masculinities and Femininities in Military Communities of Practice," *International Journal of Lifelong Education* 30, no. 3 (June 2011): 331–48, https://doi.org/10.1080/02601370.2011.570871.

42. Catherine A. MacKinnon, "Difference and Dominance: On Sex Discrimination," in *Feminism Unmodified: Discourses on Life and Law* (Cambridge, MA: Harvard University Press, 1987), 44.

43. Charlsy Panzino, "Take Three Years Off: Army Expands Career Intermission Pilot Program," *Army Times*, August 7, 2017, https://www.armytimes.com/news/your-army/2017/07/09/take-three-years-off-army-expands-career-intermission-pilot-program/.

44. Tara Copp, "Carter: '1 or 2' Years More in Rank with Proposed 'Up or Out' Policy Changes," *Stars and Stripes*, June 23, 2016, https://www.stripes.com/news/carter-1-or-2-years-more-in-rank-with-proposed-up-or-out-policy-changes-1.415892#.WXDHCIqQyRt.

45. United States Department of Defense. "DoD Instruction 1327.07 Career Intermission Program (CIP) for Service Members."

46. Air Force's Personnel Center, "Career Intermission Program," accessed June 7, 2019, https://www.afpc.af.mil/Career-Management/CIP/.

47. Scott Maucione, "Why Are So Few Troops Signing Up for One of DoD's Most Flexible Personnel Pilot Programs?," *Federal News Network*, April 3, 2018, https://federalnewsnetwork.com/defense-main/2018/04/taking-a-break-why-one-of-dods-flagship-personnel-programs-is-struggling/.

48. Maucione, "Why Are So Few Troops Signing Up."

49. United States Department of Defense, "DoD Instruction 1327.07 Career Intermission Program (CIP) for Service Members," October 18, 2018, https://www.google.com/url?sa=t&rct=j&q=&esrc=s&source=web&cd=5&ved=2ahUKEwjI_8Pj1tXiAhXFg-AKHXg-.

50. Maucione, "Why Are So Few Troops Signing Up?"

51. Ashley Rowland, "Military Bases Struggle with Breast-Feeding Policies," *Stars and Stripes*, June 18, 2015, https://www.stripes.com/news/pacific/military-bases-struggle-with-breast-feeding-policies-1.352989.

52. Mom2Momglobal, Breastfeeding in Combat Boots, "Military Policies," accessed June 6, 2019, https://www.mom2momglobal.org/breastfeeding-in-combat-boots.

53. Frank J. Barrett, "The Organizational Construction of Hegemonic Masculinity: The Case of the US Navy," *Gender, Work & Organization* 3, no. 3 (1996): 129–42.

54. Cynthia Enloe, "Beyond Steve Canyon and Rambo: Feminist Histories of Militarized Masculinity," in *Militarization of Western World*, ed. John Gillis (New Brunswick, NJ: Rutgers University Press, 1989), 119.

55. Melissa T. Brown, *Enlisting Masculinity: The Construction of Gender in US Military Recruiting Advertising during the All-Volunteer Force* (New York: Oxford University Press, 2012), 185.

CHAPTER 3. HYPERPLANNING PREGNANCIES

1. Department of the Navy, "OPNAV Instruction 6000.1C," June 14, 2007, http://doni.daps.dla.mil/Directives/06000%20Medical%20and%20Dental%20Services/06-00%20General%20Medical%20and%20Dental%20Support%20Services/6000.1C.PDF.

2. Kelsey Holt et al., "Unintended Pregnancy and Contraceptive Use among Women in the US Military: A Systematic Literature Review," *Military Medicine* 176, no. 9 (2011): 1056–1064; Genevra Pittman, "Unintended Pregnancies on the Rise in Servicewomen," Reuters, January 24, 2013,

http://www.reuters.com/article/2013/01/24/us-pregnancies-service woman-idUSBRE90N1B820130124; Catherine Pearson, "Unplanned Pregnancies Among Women In Military High, Rising," *Huffington Post*, January 23, 2013, sec. Women, http://www.huffingtonpost.com/2013/01/23/pregnant-military-unplanned-women_n_2534873.html. This is the most recent data available regarding unintended pregnancies in the military.

3. R. Lee Biggs et al., "The Impact of Pregnancy on the Individual and Military Organization: A Postpartum Active Duty Survey," *Military Medicine* 174, no. 1 (2009): 61–75; M. R. Duke and G. M. Ames, "Challenges of Contraceptive Use and Pregnancy Prevention Among Women in the U.S. Navy," *Qualitative Health Research* 18, no. 2 (February 1, 2008): 244–53, https://doi.org/10.1177/1049732307312305; Mary Ann Evans and Leora Rosen, "Pregnancy Planning and the Impact on Work Climate, Psychological Well-Being, and Work Effort in the Military," *Journal of Occupational Health Psychology* 2, no. 4 (1997): 353; Meg Gerrard, Frederick X. Gibbons, and Teddy D. Warner, "Effects of Reviewing Risk-Relevant Behavior on Perceived Vulnerability among Women Marines," *Health Psychology* 10, no. 3 (1991): 173; Holt et al., "Unintended Pregnancy and Contraceptive Use"; Janet C. Jacobson and Jeffrey T. Jensen, "A Policy of Discrimination," *Women's Health Issues* 21, no. 4 (July 2011): 255–58, https://doi.org/10.1016/j.whi.2011.03.008; Laurie A. Kwolek, Cristobal S. Berry-Caban, and Sean F. Thomas, "Pregnant Soldiers Participation in Physical Training: A Descriptive Study," *Military Medicine* 176, no. 8 (2011): 926–31; Patricia A. Thomas and Maria D. Thomas, "Effects of Sex, Marital Status, and Parental Status on Absenteeism among Navy Enlisted Personnel," *Military Psychology* 6, no. 2 (1994): 95–108.

4. Biggs et al., "The Impact of Pregnancy"; Evans and Rosen, "Pregnancy Planning and the Impact on Work Climate"; Holt et al., "Unintended Pregnancy and Contraceptive Use."

5. Holt et al., "Unintended Pregnancy and Contraceptive Use." There are significantly more enlisted personnel than officers. Enlisted servicemembers may join the military immediately after high school and are lower in rank. An enlisted servicemember can never outrank an officer of any level. The most basic requirement for an officer is a bachelor's degree. Officers serve in managerial roles and receive better compensation.

6. Ryan J. Heitmann et al., "Unintended Pregnancy in the Military Health Care System: Who Is Really at Risk?" *Military Medicine* 181, no. 10 (October 2016): 1370–74, https://doi.org/10.7205/MILMED-D-16-00003.

7. Pittman, "Unintended Pregnancies on the Rise in Servicewomen"; Megan D. McFarlane, "U.S. Military Policy and the Discursive Construction of Servicewomen's Bodies," ProQuest Dissertations Publishing, 2015; Kate Grindlay, "A Guide to Birth Control When You're in the Military," *Bedsider*, November 8, 2016, https://www.bedsider.org/features/967-a-guide-to-birth-control-when-you-re-in-the-military.

8. Grindlay, "A Guide to Birth Control When You're in the Military."

9. Duke and Ames, "Challenges of Contraceptive Use," 245.

10. Kate Grindlay and Daniel Grossman, "Contraception Access and Use among U.S. Servicewomen during Deployment," *Contraception* 87, no. 2 (2013): 162–69, https://doi.org/10.1016/j.contraception.2012.09.019.

11. Stephanie Russell-Kraft, "The Double Standard of Military Pregnancy: What Contraceptive Access Won't Fix," *Rewire News*, August 2, 2016, https://rewire.news/article/2016/08/02/double-standard-military-pregnancy-what-contraceptive-access-wont-fix/.

12. Howard P. "Buck" McKeon, "National Defense Authorization Act for Fiscal Year 2013," Pub. L. No. H.R.4310.EAS (2012), http://thomas.loc.gov/cgi-bin/query/D?c112:6:./temp/~c112P3QZ32::; Laura Bassett, "Military Abortion Amendment Is Included in Final Defense Bill," *Huffington Post*, December 18, 2012, http://www.huffingtonpost.com/2012/12/18/military-abortion-amendment_n_2324969.html.

13. McFarlane, "U.S. Military Policy and the Discursive Construction"; Megan D. McFarlane, "Circuits of Discipline: Intensified Responsibilization and the Double Bind of Pregnancy in the U.S. Military," *Women's Studies in Communication* 41, no. 1 (January 2, 2018): 22–41, https://doi.org/10.1080/07491409.2017.1419525.

14. Kate Grindlay and Daniel Grossman, "Unintended Pregnancy among Active-Duty Women in the United States Military, 2008," *Obstetrics & Gynecology* 121, no. 2, PART 1 (2013): 241–46.

15. Kathryn L. Ponder and Melissa Nothnagle, "Damage Control: Unintended Pregnancy in the United States Military," *Journal of Law, Medicine & Ethics* 38, no. 2 (2010): 386–95.

16. Biggs et al., "The Impact of Pregnancy," 64.

17. Jennifer Hickes Lundquist and Herbert L. Smith, "Family Formation among Women in the US Military: Evidence from the NLSY," *Journal of Marriage and Family* 67, no. 1 (2005): 1–13.

18. Holt et al., "Unintended Pregnancy and Contraceptive Use," 1060.

19. Erving Goffman, *Stigma: Notes on the Management of Spoiled Identity* (New York: Simon and Schuster, 1963), 1.

20. Katie Margavio Striley, "The Stigma of Excellence and the Dialectic of (Perceived) Superiority and Inferiority: Exploring Intellectually Gifted Adolescents' Experiences of Stigma," *Communication Studies* 65, no. 2 (2014): 139–53, http://dx.doi.org/10.1080/10510974.2013.851726.

21. Biggs et al., "The Impact of Pregnancy"; Jacobson and Jensen, "A Policy of Discrimination."

22. Evans and Rosen, "Pregnancy Planning and the Impact on Work Climate."

23. Part of the PT test also includes a body fat test. Servicewomen are exempt from PT tests while pregnant, and for at least six months postpartum. Naval Physical Readiness Program, "Guide 8: Managing Physical Fitness Assessment Records for Pregnant Servicewomen," U.S. Navy, 2016, http://www.public.navy.mil/bupers-npc/support/21st_Century_Sailor/physical/Documents/Guide%208-%20Managing%20PFA%20Records%20for%20Pregnant%20Service%20Women%202016%20(F).pdf.

24. Connie Bullis and Karen Rohrbauck Stout, "Organizational Socialization: A Feminist Standpoint Approach," in *Rethinking Organizational and Managerial Communication from Feminist Perspectives*, ed. Patrice M. Buzzanell (Thousand Oaks, CA: SAGE, 2000).

25. McFarlane, "Circuits of Discipline."

26. Michel Foucault, *Discipline and Punish: The Birth of the Prison*, 2nd ed. (New York: Vintage, 1995).

27. See chapter 1 for more details.

28. Suzy D'Enbeau and Patrice M. Buzzanell, "Efficiencies of Pregnancy Management," in *Culture of Efficiency: Technology in Everyday Life*, ed. Sharon Kleinman (New York: Peter Lang, 2009), 4.

29. Department of the Navy, "OPNAV Instruction 6000.1C," 201.c.(1). OPNAV 6001.C was the Instruction that servicewomen used at the time of the interviews. The Instruction has been updated to OPNAV 6001.D, and this language is no longer included.

30. Navy Office of Women's Policy, "Women's Policy," Department of the Navy, accessed February 27, 2014, http://www.public.navy.mil/bupers-npc/organization/bupers/WomensPolicy/Documents/Women%27s%20Policy%20Handout.pdf. In early 2017, the Navy Office of Women's Policy was dissolved. I had accessed their documents, and saved some, prior to 2017, but they are not accessible online anymore. However, since 1951, the Defense Advisory Committee on Women in the Services (DACOWITS) has been a federal advisory committee that works directly

for the secretary of defense. Additionally, each diversity office within the military services has a gender policy advisor.

31. Department of the Navy, "OPNAV Instruction 6000.1C."

32. Joanne Martin, "Deconstructing Organizational Taboos: The Suppression of Gender Conflict in Organizations," *Organization Science* 1, no. 4 (1990), 347, http://www.jstor.org/stable/pdf/2634968.pdf.

33. For an in-depth analysis of the science behind the fertility clock and risky pregnancies, see Robin E. Jensen, *Infertility: Tracing the History of a Transformative Term* (University Park: Pennsylvania State University Press, 2016).

34. Biggs et al., "The Impact of Pregnancy"; Jacobson and Jensen, "A Policy of Discrimination."

35. Adam Sonfield, Kinsey Hasstedt, and Rachel Benson Gold, *Moving Forward: Family Planning in the Era of Health Reform*, Guttmacher Institute, January 27, 2016, https://www.guttmacher.org/report/moving-forward-family-planning-era-health-reform. The researchers also found that of unintended pregnancies, 5 percent are "women who used their method perfectly but who experienced method failure."

36. Duke and Ames, "Challenges of Contraceptive Use."

37. Duke and Ames, "Challenges of Contraceptive Use," 245.

38. Rebecca Todd Peters, *Trust Women: A Progressive Christian Argument for Reproductive Justice* (Boston: Beacon Press, 2018), 54.

39. Department of the Navy, "OPNAV Instruction 6000.1C," secs. 104, 105(d).

40. Specifically, the Instructions say, "In-Vitro Fertilization (IVF). Servicewomen undergoing infertility treatment with IVF are required to inform their command with a letter from their HCP that should include the duration of the treatment, the potential dates for minor procedures such as oocyte retrieval and embryo transfer, so that possible duty limitations and TAD may be anticipated. During the actual IVF cycles, servicewomen will be exempt from participating in the PFA and BCA to better ensure IVF success. Women who participate in IVF programs are more likely to gain weight due to numerous hormone treatments and must limit physical activity to increase IVF success rates and prevent additional IVF treatments. When IVF treatment results in a successful pregnancy, the provisions of this policy will pertain. If the IVF treatment is unsuccessful, the servicewoman will be expected to participate fully in the PFA and BCA in 30 days." Department of the Navy, "OPNAV Instruction 6000.1C," sec. 207.

41. Atwood D. Gaines and Robbie Davis-Floyd, "Biomedicine," in *Encyclopedia of Medical Anthropology: Health and Illness in the World's Cultures*, ed. Carol R. Ember and Melvin Ember, vol. 1 (New York: Kluwer Academic/Plenum Publishers, 2004).

CHAPTER 4. PERFORMING MACHO MATERNITY

1. Lolita C. Baldor, "US Navy Triples Paid Maternity Leave in Effort to Attract Women," Military.com, July 3, 2015, http://www.military.com/daily-news/2015/07/03/us-navy-triple-paid-maternity-leave-in-effort-to-attract-women.html.

2. Iris Marion Young, *On Female Body Experience: "Throwing Like a Girl" and Other Essays* (New York: Oxford University Press, 2005), 47.

3. Stephanie Gutmann, "Sex and the Soldier," *The New Republic*, February 24, 1997, 21.

4. Elizabeth C. Britt, *Conceiving Normalcy: Rhetoric, Law, and the Double Binds of Infertility* (Tuscaloosa: University of Alabama Press, 2001), 33.

5. Young, *On Female Body Experience*, 57.

6. Michel Foucault, *The History of Sexuality, Vol. 1: An Introduction*, trans. Robert Hurley (New York: Vintage, 1976), 104.

7. Marouf Hasian Jr., "The 'Hysterical' Emily Hobhouse and Boer War Concentration Camp Controversy," *Western Journal of Communication* 67, no. 2 (Spring 2003): 138–163, https://doi.org/10.1080/10570310309374764.

8. Amy Koerber, *From Hysteria to Hormones: A Rhetorical History* (University Park: Pennsylvania State University Press, 2018), 168.

9. Department of the Navy, "OPNAV Instruction 6000.1C," sec. 101(e)(3), June 14, 2007, http://doni.daps.dla.mil/Directives/06000%20Medical%20and%20Dental%20Services/06-00%20General%20Medical%20and%20Dental%20Support%20Services/6000.1C.PDF.

10. Anne-Marie Slaughter, *Unfinished Business: Women Men Work Family*, reprint ed. (New York: Random House, 2016), 31.

11. Carol Tarvis, *The Mismeasure of Woman: Why Women Are Not the Better Sex, the Inferior Sex, or the Opposite Sex* (New York: Touchstone, 1992), 119.

12. Patrice M. Buzzanell and Laura L. Ellingson, "Contesting Narratives of Workplace Maternity," in *Narratives, Health, and Healing: Communication Theory, Research, and Practice*, ed. Lynn M. Harter,

Phyllis M. Japp, and Christina S. Beck (Mahwah, NJ: Lawrence Erlbaum, 2005), 282.

13. Sarah Kornfield, "Pregnant Discourse: 'Having It All' While Domestic and Potentially Disabled," *Women's Studies in Communication* 37, no. 2 (May 4, 2014): 192, https://doi.org/10.1080/07491409.2014.911233.

14. Naval Physical Readiness Program, "Guide 8: Managing Physical Fitness Assessment Records for Pregnant Servicewomen," U.S. Navy, 2016, 8, http://www.public.navy.mil/bupers-npc/support/21st_Century_Sailor/physical/Documents/Guide%208-%20Managing%20PFA%20Records%20for%20Pregnant%20Service%20Women%202016%20(F).pdf; Department of the Navy, "OPNAV Instruction 6000.1C."

15. Alexandra G. Murphy, "The Dialectical Gaze: Exploring the Subject-Object Tension in the Performances of Women Who Strip," *Journal of Contemporary Ethnography* 32, no. 3 (June 1, 2003): 305–35. https://doi.org/10.1177/0891241603032003003.

16. Bethanee Bemis, "Pregnant in Uniform," National Museum of American History, September 26, 2011, https://americanhistory.si.edu/blog/2011/09/pregnant-in-uniform.html.

17. Rebecca Todd Peters, *Trust Women: A Progressive Christian Argument for Reproductive Justice* (Boston: Beacon Press, 2018).

18. Ellen D. Hodnet, "Continuity of Caregivers for Care during Pregnancy and Childbirth," *Cochrane Database of Systematic Reviews*, no. 1 (2000), https://doi.org/10.1002/14651858.CD000062; World Health Organization, "WHO Recommendation on Midwife-Led Continuity of Care during Pregnancy," November 1, 2016, https://extranet.who.int/rhl/topics/improving-health-system-performance/implementation-strategies/who-recommendation-midwife-led-continuity-care-during-pregnancy.

19. Navy Personnel Command, "Pregnancy and Parenthood," United States Navy, accessed July 18, 2109, https://www.public.navy.mil/bupers-npc/support/21st_Century_Sailor/PregnancyParenthood/Pages/default.aspx.

20. Michel Foucault, *Discipline & Punish: The Birth of the Prison*, 2nd ed. (New York: Vintage, 1995).

21. Rebecca J. Meisenbach et al., "'They Allowed': Pentadic Mapping of Women's Maternity Leave Discourse as Organizational Rhetoric," *Communication Monographs* 75, no. 1 (March 1, 2008): 1–24, https://doi.org/10.1080/03637750801952727.

22. Janet Smithson and Elizabeth H. Stokoe, "Discourses of Work-Life Balance: Negotiating 'Genderblind' Terms in Organizations," *Gender, Work & Organization* 12, no. 2 (2005): 147–68.

23. Smithson and Stokoe, "Discourses of Work–Life Balance," 160, 164.

24. Navy Personnel Command, "Pregnancy FAQs," January 18, 2017, http://www.public.navy.mil/bupers-npc/organization/bupers/WomensPolicy/Pages/FAQs-Women'sPolicy.aspx.

25. Patrice M. Buzzanell, "Reframing the Glass Ceiling as a Socially Constructed Process: Implications for Understanding and Change," *Communication Monographs* 62 (1995): 334.

CHAPTER 5. NEGOTIATING POSTPARTUM POLICIES

1. Joan Acker, "Hierarchies, Jobs, Bodies: A Theory of Gendered Organizations," *Gender & Society* 4, no. 2 (June 1, 1990): 139–58, https://doi.org/10.1177/089124390004002002; Paaige K. Turner and Kristen Norwood, "Unbounded Motherhood: Embodying a Good Working Mother Identity," *Management Communication Quarterly* 27, no. 3 (2013): 396–424.

2. Karen Lee Ashcraft, "Managing Maternity Leave: A Qualitative Analysis of Temporary Executive Succession," *Administrative Science Quarterly* 44 (1999): 244.

3. Rosi Braidotti, "Mothers, Monsters, and Machines," in *Writing on the Body: Female Embodiment and Feminist Theory*, ed. Katie Conboy, Nadia Medina, and Sarah Stanbury (New York: Columbia University Press, 1997), 59–79.

4. Turner and Norwood, "Unbounded Motherhood"; Ashcraft, "Managing Maternity Leave."

5. Smithson and Stokoe, "Discourses of Work–Life Balance: Negotiating 'Genderblind' Terms in Organizations," *Gender, Work & Organization* 12, no. 2 (2005): 147–68.

6. Smithson and Stokoe, "Discourses of Work–Life Balance, 148.

7. Mary Blair-Loy, "Cultural Constructions of Family Schemas: The Case of Women Finance Executives," *Gender & Society* 15, no. 5 (2001): 706.

8. Lindal Buchanan, *Rhetorics of Motherhood* (Carbondale: Southern Illinois University Press, 2013); D. Lynn O'Brien Hallstein, "Introduction to Mothering Rhetorics," *Women's Studies in Communication* 40, no. 1 (2017): 1–10, http://dx.doi.org/10.1080/07491409.2017.1280326.

9. Adrienne Rich, *Of Woman Born: Motherhood as Experience and Institution* (New York: W. W. Norton & Company, 1995).

10. Diane Eyer, *Motherguilt: How Our Culture Blames Mothers for What's Wrong with Society* (New York: Random House, 1996), 233; Buchanan, *Rhetorics of Motherhood*, 5.

11. Sharon Hays, *The Cultural Contradictions of Motherhood* (New Haven, CT: Yale University Press, 1996).

12. Susan Douglas and Meredith Michaels, *The Mommy Myth: The Idealization of Motherhood and How It Has Undermined All Women* (New York: Free Press, 2004).

13. O'Brien Hallstein, "Introduction to Mothering Rhetorics."

14. Natalie Fixmer-Oraiz, *Homeland Maternity: US Security Culture and the New Reproductive Regime* (Urbana: University of Illinois Press, 2019).

15. Mack, "Disciplining Mommy: Rhetorics of Reproduction in Contemporary Maternity Culture," PhD diss. The University of Texas at Austin, 2013, 9, http://repositories.lib.utexas.edu/bitstream/ handle/2152/21299 /MACK-DISSERTATION-2013.pdf?sequence=1.

16. Mack, "Disciplining Mommy"; Douglas and Michaels, *The Mommy Myth*; O'Brien Hallstein, "Introduction to Mothering Rhetorics."

17. D. Lynn O'Brien Hallstein, "Silences and Choice: The Legacies of White Second Wave Feminism in the New Professoriate," *Women's Studies in Communication* 31, no. 2 (July 2008): 143–50, https://doi.org/10.1080/07491409 .2008.10162526. See also Douglas and Michaels, *The Mommy Myth*.

18. Eyer, *Motherguilt*, 3.

19. Jessica L. Collett, "What Kind of Mother Am I?: Impression Management and the Social Construction of Motherhood," *Symbolic Interaction* 28, no. 3 (August 2005): 327–47, https://doi.org/10.1525/si.2005.28 .3.327.

20. O'Brien Hallstein, "Silences and Choice."

21. Eyer, *Motherguilt*.

22. O'Brien Hallstein, "Introduction to Mothering Rhetorics," 3.

23. Patrice M. Buzzanell and Meina Liu, "Struggling with Maternity Leave Policies and Practices: A Poststructuralist Feminist Analysis of Gendered Organizing," *Journal of Applied Communication Research* 33, no. 1 (February 2005): 1–25, https://doi.org/10.1080/0090988042000318495; Patrice M. Buzzanell et al., "The Good *Working* Mother: Managerial Women's Sensemaking and Feelings about Work–Family Issues," *Communication Studies* 56, no. 3 (January 2005): 261–85, https://doi.org/10.1080 /10510970500181389; Turner and Norwood, "Unbounded Motherhood."

24. Hays, *The Cultural Contradictions of Motherhood*; Anne Machung, "Talking Career, Thinking Job: Gender Differences in Career and Family Expectations of Berkeley Seniors," *Feminist Studies* 15, no. 1 (1989): 35, https://doi.org/10.2307/3177817. For a discussion of the reasons that both

have intensified concurrently, see Douglas and Michaels, *The Mommy Myth*, 9–11.

25. Joanne Martin, "Deconstructing Organizational Taboos: The Suppression of Gender Conflict in Organizations," *Organization Science* 1, no. 4 (1990), http://www.jstor.org/stable/pdf/2634968.pdf.

26. Paaige K. Turner and Kristen Norwood, "The Elephant in the Room: Negotiating Visible Pregnancy in Job Interviews," *Women & Language* 37, no. 1 (2014): 43.

27. Deirdre D. Johnston and Debra H. Swanson, "Cognitive Acrobatics in the Construction of Worker–Mother Identity," *Sex Roles* 57, nos. 5–6 (August 21, 2007): 447–59, https://doi.org/10.1007/s11199-007-9267-4.

28. Turner and Norwood, "Unbounded Motherhood." The terms *bounded* and *unbounded* relate to breastfeeding. As Turner and Norwood explain, "In the past, mothers who did not wish to breastfeed would bind their breasts to stop the production of milk. This can be seen as an apt metaphor for many women today who combine breastfeeding and paid labor. Breastfeeding workers describe suppressing breastfeeding practices at work to limit disruptions and maintain credibility as good workers. The binding of motherhood at work creates difficulties that may contribute to early cessation of breastfeeding. In effect, women's bodies, in addition to their identities, are bound by the material and discursive separation of and tension between motherhood and work. However, women may be finding ways to materially negotiate this tension, just as they find ways to discursively manage it" (p. 397). See also Deborah Payne and David A. Nicholls, "Managing Breastfeeding and Work: A Foucauldian Secondary Analysis: Managing Breastfeeding and Work," *Journal of Advanced Nursing* 66, no. 8 (June 16, 2010): 1810–18, https://doi.org/10.1111/j.1365-2648.2009.05156.x.

29. An example of bounded motherhood in the U.S. military is the uniform. See chapter 4 for more discussion.

30. Douglas and Michaels, *The Mommy Myth*; Rebecca Todd Peters, *Trust Women: A Progressive Christian Argument for Reproductive Justice* (Boston: Beacon Press, 2018).

31. Buzzanell et al., "The Good *Working* Mother," 252.

32. Linda Martin Alcoff, "Identities: Modern and Postmodern," in *Identities: Race, Class, Gender, and Nationality* (Malden, MA: Blackwell Publishing, 2003), 1–8; Jennifer M. Heisler and Jennifer Butler Ellis, "Motherhood and the Construction of 'Mommy Identity': Messages

about Motherhood and Face Negotiation," *Communication Quarterly* 56, no. 4 (November 19, 2008): 445–67, https://doi.org/10.1080/01463370802448246.

33. Alice Truong, "When Google Increased the Length of Paid Maternity Leave, the Rate New Mothers Quit Dropped by 50%," *Quartz*, January 28, 2016, https://qz.com/604723/when-google-increased-paid-maternity-leave-the-rate-at-which-new-mothers-quit-dropped-50/.

34. Sharon Lerner, "The Real War on Families: Why the U.S. Needs Paid Leave Now," *In These Times*, August 18, 2015, http://inthesetimes.com/article/18151/the-real-war-on-families.

35. Amanda Lenhart, Haley Swenson, and Brigid Schulte, "Lifting the Barriers to Paid Family and Medical Leave for Men in the United States," New America, accessed June 23, 2020, http://newamerica.org/better-life-lab/reports/lifting-barriers-paid-family-and-medical-leave-men-united-states/.

36. Jackie Wattles, "Is It Time for Universal Paid Family Leave?," CNN, July 31, 2017, https://money.cnn.com/2017/07/31/news/economy/kirsten-gillibrand-family-act/index.html.

37. For example, see Eyer, *Motherguilt*. In terms of bipartisan support, Senator Kirsten Gillibrand (D-New York) has introduced a paid family leave bill every year for many years, and in 2017, President Donald Trump and his daughter, Ivanka Trump, each supported paid family and maternity leave, respectively. See Heather Long, "Did Donald Trump Endorse Paid FAMILY Leave?" CNNMoney, March 6, 2017, https://money.cnn.com/2017/03/06/news/economy/donald-trump-paid-family-leave/index.html.; Wattles, "Is It Time for Universal Paid Family Leave?"

38. Long, "Did Donald Trump Endorse Paid FAMILY Leave?"; Jon Greenberg, "Yes, the United States Is the Only Industrialized Nation without Paid Family Leave," *PolitiFact*, July 25, 2016, https://www.politifact.com/truth-o-meter/statements/2016/jul/25/kirsten-gillibrand/yes-us-only-industrialized-nation-without-paid-fam/.

39. Wattles, "Is It Time for Universal Paid Family Leave?"

40. Jennifer Ludden, "FMLA Not Really Working for Many Employees," NPR.org, February 5, 2013, https://www.npr.org/2013/02/05/171078451/fmla-not-really-working-for-many-employees.

41. Ray Mabus, "Video: SECNAV Ray Mabus Speech on Navy Personnel Changes," *USNI News* (blog), May 15, 2015, https://news.usni.org/2015/05/15/video-secnav-ray-mabus-speech-on-navy-personnel-changes.

42. U.S. Navy, "SECNAV Announces Personnel Initiatives," Navy Live, May 13, 2015, http://navylive.dodlive.mil/2015/05/13/secnav-announces-personnel-initiatives/.

43. Mark D. Faram, "SECNAV Orders Review of Fitness, Advancement Changes," *Navy Times*, June 12, 2015, para. 43, https://www.navytimes.com/story/military/careers/2015/06/12/navy-personnel-initiatives-mabus-alnav/71017838/.

44. Bryant Jordan, "US Navy Triples Maternity Leave to 18 Weeks for Sailors and Marines," Military.com, August 6, 2015, para. 2 http://www.military.com/daily-news/2015/08/06/us-navy-triples-maternity-leave-to-18-weeks-for-sailors-marines.html.

45. Meghann Myers, "Navy Rolls Back Maternity Leave from 18 to 12 Weeks," *Navy Times*, February 25, 2015, https://www.navytimes.com/story/military/2016/02/25/navy-rolls-back-maternity-leave-18-12-weeks/80939818/.

46. Faram, "SECNAV Orders Review of Fitness"; Ray Mabus, "DoN Talent Management Address to the Brigade of Midshipmen," Annapolis, MD, May 13, 2015, 4, https://news.usni.org/2015/05/15/video-secnav-ray-mabus-speech-on-navy-personnel-changes. Currently, servicewomen comprise about 17 percent of the military according to Reynolds and Shendruk, "Demographics of the U.S. Military," Council on Foreign Relations, April 24, 2018, https://www.cfr.org/article/demographics-us-military. This goal for a critical mass of women is supported by research. See Paula A. Johnson, Sheila E. Widnall, and Frazier F. Benya, eds., *Sexual Harassment of Women: Climate, Culture, and Consequences in Academic Sciences, Engineering, and Medicine* (Washington, DC: The National Academies Press, 2018). They note that researchers have found the critical mass of women in an organization to be 30 percent.

47. Office of the Chief of Information, "SECNAV Announces New Maternity Leave Policy," para. 3.

48. Schwartz brought up this point in 1989 when discussing why women often fail to advance. The low retention rate of women meant that all of the money on training was ultimately wasted, which made many employers hesitant to train women. Schwartz, "Management Women and the New Facts of Life."

49. Office of the Chief of Information, "SECNAV Announces New Maternity Leave Policy," *America's Navy*, July 2, 2015, para. 5, http://www.navy.mil/submit/display.asp?story_id=87987.

50. Office of the Chief of Information, "SECNAV Announces New Maternity Leave Policy," para. 6.

51. Lolita C. Baldor, "US Navy Triples Paid Maternity Leave in Effort to Attract Women," Military.com, July 3, 2015, http://www.military.com/daily-news/2015/07/03/us-navy-triple-paid-maternity-leave-in-effort-to-attract-women.html.

52. Douglas and Michaels, *The Mommy Myth*.

53. Collett, "What Kind of Mother Am I?"; Heisler and Ellis, "Motherhood and the Construction of 'Mommy Identity.'"

54. Machung, "Talking Career, Thinking Job."

55. Department of the Navy, OPNAV (N130), "MILPERSMAN 1050-435: Maternity Leave," November 18, 2016, https://www.public.navy.mil/bupers-npc/reference/milpersman/1000/1000General/Documents/1050-435.pdf.

56. Office of the Chief of Information, "SECNAV Announces New Maternity Leave Policy," para. 7. And, if a woman had another pregnancy and an additional child in that year, the leave reset to eighteen more weeks. See Meghann Myers, "Navy Triples Maternity Leave for Sailors, Starting Now," *Navy Times*, August 5, 2015, para. 7, https://www.navytimes.com/story/military/2015/08/05/navy-triples-maternity-leave-sailors-starting-now/31168645/.

57. Myers, "Navy Triples Maternity Leave," para. 5.

58. Myers, "Navy Triples Maternity Leave," para. 6; Truong, "When Google Increased the Length of Paid Maternity Leave, the Rate New Mothers Quit Dropped by 50%"; in fact, many tech companies have been changing their leave policies. See Jay Moye, "Paid Leave for All Parents: Millennial Employees Drive Coke's New Parental Benefits Policy," The Coca-Cola Company, April 11, 2016, https://www.coca-colacompany.com/stories/paid-leave-for-all-parents--millennial-employees-drive-cokes-new/; Alicia Adamczyk, "These Are the Companies with the Best Parental Leave Policies," *Money*, November 4, 2015, http://time.com/money/4098469/paid-parental-leave-google-amazon-apple-facebook/.

59. Myers, "Navy Triples Maternity Leave."

60. Jordan, "US Navy Triples Maternity Leave to 18 Weeks for Sailors and Marines," para. 6.

61. Baldor, "US Navy Triples Paid Maternity Leave in Effort to Attract Women."

62. Reynolds and Shendruk, "Demographics of the U.S. Military."

63. *Morning Edition*, "Navy, Marine Corps Now Offer 18 Weeks of Maternity Leave," NPR, July 8, 2015, http://www.npr.org/2015/07/08/421083589/navy-marine-corps-now-offer-18-weeks-of-maternity-leave.

64. Amy Bushatz, "Pentagon Sets Maternity Leave at 12 Weeks for All Services," Military.com, January 28, 2016 para. 3, http://www.military.com/daily-news/2016/01/28/maternity-leave-slashed-for-sailors-marines.html.

65. Bushatz, para. 5.

66. Courtney Kube and Jim Miklaszewski, "Military to Announce Changes to Maternity Leave Policy," NBC News, January 28, 2016, http://www.nbcnews.com/news/us-news/military-announce-changes-maternity-leave-policy-n506006.

67. Kube and Miklaszewski.

68. Myers, "Navy Rolls Back Maternity Leave from 18 to 12 Weeks."

69. Peters, *Trust Women*.

70. Mayo Clinic Staff, "High-Risk Pregnancy: Know What to Expect," Mayo Clinic, February 21, 2018, http://www.mayoclinic.org/healthy-lifestyle/pregnancy-week-by-week/in-depth/high-risk-pregnancy/art-20047012.

71. Myers, "Navy Rolls Back Maternity Leave from 18 to 12 Weeks."

72. Tara Copp, "Carter: '1 or 2' Years More in Rank with Proposed 'Up or Out' Policy Changes," *Stars and Stripes*, June 23, 2016, https://www.stripes.com/news/carter-1-or-2-years-more-in-rank-with-proposed-up-or-out-policy-changes-1.415892#.WXDHCIqQyRt.

73. Nikki C. Townsley and Kirsten J. Broadfoot, "Care, Career, and Academe: Heeding the Calls of a New Professoriate," *Women's Studies in Communication* 31, no. 2 (Summer 2008): 133–42, https://doi.org/10.1080/07491409.2008.10162525.

74. Myers, "Navy Rolls Back Maternity Leave from 18 to 12 Weeks."

75. It should be noted that due to the nature of snowball sampling methods, as well as the two different phases of interviews, this chapter contains primarily insights from officers, rather than enlisted servicewomen.

76. Joanna Weiss, "Chris Cuomo, Stay in Bed," Politico, April 6, 2020, https://www.politico.com/news/magazine/2020/04/06/chris-cuomo-stay-in-bed-167297.

77. Incidentally, many men in the military and elsewhere often refuse parental leave to avoid being seen in this way. See Megan McFarlane, "Circuits of Discipline: Intensified Responsibilization and the Double Bind of Pregnancy in the U.S. Military," *Women's Studies in Communication*

41, no. 1 (January 2, 2018): 22–41, https://doi.org/10.1080/07491409.2017.1419525.

78. Buzzanell and Liu, "Struggling with Maternity Leave Policies and Practices."

79. Buzzanell et al., "The Good *Working* Mother," 263.

80. Douglas and Michaels, *The Mommy Myth*, 7.

81. See chapter 3 for further discussion.

82. Anne-Marie Slaughter, *Unfinished Business: Women Men Work Family*, reprint ed. (New York: Random House, 2016), 16.

83. O'Brien Hallstein, "Silences and Choice."

84. Rebecca J. Meisenbach et al., "'They Allowed': Pentadic Mapping of Women's Maternity Leave Discourse as Organizational Rhetoric," *Communication Monographs* 75, no. 1 (March 1, 2008): 1–24, https://doi.org/10.1080/03637750801952727.

85. Turner and Norwood, "Unbounded Motherhood"; Koerber, *Breast or Bottle?: Contemporary Controversies in Infant-Feeding Policy and Practice* (Columbia: University of South Carolina Press, 2013); Mack, "Disciplining Mommy."

86. Koerber, *Breast or Bottle?*, 132.

87. Joan B. Wolf, *Is Breast Best?: Taking on the Breastfeeding Experts and the New High Stakes of Motherhood* (New York: New York University Press, 2010).

88. Turner and Norwood, "Unbounded Motherhood."

89. I am using Navy policies in this section because a majority of the servicewomen interviewed who responded to this topic were in the Navy.

90. Department of the Navy, "OPNAV Instruction 6000.1C," June 14, 2007, 39–40, http://doni.daps.dla.mil/Directives/06000%20Medical%20and%20Dental%20Services/06-00%20General%20Medical%20and%20Dental%20Support%20Services/6000.1C.PDF.

91. Mack, "Disciplining Mommy," 100.

92. Department of the Navy, "OPNAV Instruction 6000.1C."

93. Paaige K. Turner and Kristen Norwood, "'I Had the Luxury . . .': Organizational Breastfeeding Support as Privatized Privilege," *Human Relations* 67, no. 7 (July 2014): 850, https://doi.org/10.1177/0018726713507730; Payne and Nicholls, "Managing Breastfeeding and Work," 1811.

94. Department of the Navy, "OPNAV Instruction 6000.1C," sec. 201(5).

95. Turner and Norwood, "Unbounded Motherhood," 401.

96. Turner and Norwood, "Unbounded Motherhood," 397.

97. Payne and Nicholls, "Managing Breastfeeding and Work."

98. Koerber, *Breast or Bottle?*

99. Leila Schochet, "The Child Care Crisis Is Keeping Women out of the Workforce," Center for American Progress, March 28, 2019, https://www.americanprogress.org/issues/early-childhood/reports/2019/03/28/467488/child-care-crisis-keeping-women-workforce/.

100. Kids Count Data Center, "Children under Age 6 with All Available Parents in the Labor Force," The Annie E. Casey Foundation Kids Count Data Center, October 2018, https://datacenter.kidscount.org/data/Tables/5057-children-under-age-6-with-all-available-parents-in-the-labor-force.

101. Leila Schochet and Rasheed Malik, "2 Million Parents Forced to Make Career Sacrifices Due to Problems with Child Care," Center for American Progress, September 13, 2017, https://www.americanprogress.org/issues/early-childhood/news/2017/09/13/438838/2-million-parents-forced-make-career-sacrifices-due-problems-child-care/. This problem has only intensified during the COVID-19 pandemic, causing what many have called a "Shesession," as women are dropping out of the labor market much faster than men due to losing their jobs or a lack of childcare. See Alisha Haridasani Gupta, "Why Some Women Call This Recession a 'Shesession,'" *New York Times*, May 9, 2020, https://www.nytimes.com/2020/05/09/us/unemployment-coronavirus-women.html.

102. Spencer Soper and Rebecca Greenfield, "Holdout Jeff Bezos Confronted by Amazon Moms Demanding Day Care," *Bloomberg*, March 4, 2019, https://www.bloomberg.com/news/articles/2019-03-04/holdout-jeff-bezos-confronted-by-amazon-moms-demanding-daycare.

103. Bridget Ansel, "Is the Cost of Childcare Driving Women out of the U.S. Workforce?" *Equitable Growth*, November 29, 2016, https://equitablegrowth.org/is-the-cost-of-childcare-driving-women-out-of-the-u-s-workforce/; Schochet, "The Child Care Crisis Is Keeping Women out of the Workforce."

104. Tracy Morison et al., "Stigma Resistance in Online Childfree Communities: The Limitations of Choice Rhetoric," *Psychology of Women Quarterly* 40, no. 2 (June 2016): 184–98, https://doi.org/10.1177/0361684315603657.

105. Hays, *The Cultural Contradictions of Motherhood*, 131 (italics in original).

106. Sara Hayden and D. Lynn O'Brien Hallstein, *Contemplating Maternity in an Era of Choice: Explorations into Discourses of Reproduction* (Lanham, MD: Lexington Books, 2010).

107. Townsley and Broadfoot, "Care, Career, and Academe."
108. Blair-Loy, "Cultural Constructions of Family Schemas."
109. Virginia McCarver, "The Rhetoric of Choice and 21st-Century Feminism: Online Conversations about Work, Family, and Sarah Palin," *Women's Studies in Communication* 34, no. 1 (May 5, 2011): 21.
110. McCarver, "The Rhetoric of Choice and 21st-Century Feminism," 22.
111. Natalie Fixmer-Oraiz, "Contemplating Homeland Maternity," *Women's Studies in Communication* 38, no. 2 (April 3, 2015): 129–34, https://doi.org/10.1080/07491409.2015.1034630; O'Brien Hallstein, "Silences and Choice"; Jennifer Borda, "Lean In or Leave before You Leave? False Dichotomies of Choice and Blame in Public Debates about Working Motherhood," in *The Mother Blame-Game*, ed. Vanessa Reimer and Sarah Sahagian (Toronto, ON: Demeter Press, 2005); McCarver, "The Rhetoric of Choice and 21st-Century Feminism"; Tasha N. Dubriwny, "Consciousness-Raising as Collective Rhetoric: The Articulation of Experience in the Redstockings' Abortion Speak-Out of 1969," *Quarterly Journal of Speech* 91, no. 4 (November 2005): 395–422, https://doi.org/10.1080/00335630500488275; Rosalind Gill, "Postfeminist Media Culture: Elements of a Sensibility," *European Journal of Cultural Studies* 10, no. 2 (2007): 147–66.
112. Eyer, *Motherguilt*; Virginia H. Mackintosh, Miriam Liss, and Holly H. Schiffrin, "Using a Quantitative Measure to Explore Intensive Mothering Ideology," in *Intensive Mothering: The Cultural Contradictions of Modern Motherhood*, ed. Linda Rose Ennis (Bradford, ON: Demeter Press, 2014), 142–59; Hays, *The Cultural Contradictions of Motherhood*; Collett, "What Kind of Mother Am I?"; D. Lynn O'Brien Hallstein, "Public Choices, Private Control: How Mediated Mom Labels Work Rhetorically to Dismantle the Politics of Choice and White Second Wave Feminist Successes," in *Contemplating Maternity in an Era of Choice: Explorations into Discourses of Reproduction*, ed. Sara Hayden and D. Lynn O'Brien Hallstein (Lanham, MD: Lexington Books, 2010), 5–26; Buzzanell et al., "The Good *Working* Mother"; McCarver, "The Rhetoric of Choice and 21st-Century Feminism"; Hayden and O'Brien Hallstein, *Contemplating Maternity in an Era of Choice*.
113. O'Brien Hallstein, "Public Choices, Private Control"; Slaughter, *Unfinished Business*.
114. Jean Y. Ko et al., "Trends in Postpartum Depressive Symptoms—27 States, 2004, 2008, and 2012," *Morbidity and Mortality Weekly Report* 66, no. 6 (2017): 153–58.

115. Sara Hayden and D. Lynn O'Brien Hallstein, "Introduction," in *Contemplating Maternity in an Era of Choice: Explorations into Discourses of Reproduction*, ed. Sara Hayden and D. Lynn O'Brien Hallstein (Lanham, MD: Lexington Books, 2010), xvi.

116. Martin, "Deconstructing Organizational Taboos."

117. Koerber, *Breast or Bottle?*, 107.

118. Karen Jowers, "More Bases Offering Extended Child Care Hours," *Military Times*, October 6, 2017, https://www.militarytimes.com/pay-benefits/2017/10/06/more-bases-offering-extended-child-care-hours/.

CHAPTER 6. REDEFINING MILITARY MATERNITY

1. Robyn Roche-Paull, "Powerful Photo of Airman Breastfeeding Shows Us What Motherhood in the Military Looks Like," Breastfeeding in Combat Boots, March 8, 2015, http://breastfeedingincombatboots.com/2015/03/powerful-photo-of-airman-breastfeeding-shows-motherhood-military-looks-like/.

2. Jade Beall Photography's Facebook Page, "Jonea Cunico," March 3, 2015, https://www.facebook.com/JadeBeallPhotography/photos/a.193038724076942.48997.193035750743906/831187540262054/?type=1.

3. Emanuella Grinberg, "Soldiers in Camo Breastfeed in Photo," CNN, September 15, 2015, https://www.cnn.com/2015/09/13/living/breastfeeding-soldiers-uniform-feat/index.html.

4. Shalah Meedya, Kathleen Fahy, and Ashley Kable, "Factors That Positively Influence Breastfeeding Duration to 6 Months: A Literature Review," *Women and Birth* 23, no. 4 (December 1, 2010): 135–45, https://doi.org/10.1016/j.wombi.2010.02.002.

5. Caroline Bologna, "Air Force Mom Breastfeeding in Uniform Is a Stunning Look at Military Motherhood," *HuffPost*, March 12, 2015, https://www.huffpost.com/entry/jonea-cunico-military-breastfeed_n_6856762.; Grinberg, "Soldiers in Camo Breastfeed in Photo."

6. Caroline Bologna, "7 Powerful Photos of Military Moms Breastfeeding in Uniform," *HuffPost*, May 12, 2016, https://www.huffpost.com/entry/7-powerful-photos-of-military-moms-breastfeeding-in-uniform_n_5730aa94e4b0bc9cb0475f14.

7. Noah Nash, "New Navy Parental Leave Policy Gives New Parents Additional Flexibility," *Navy Times*, June 22, 2018, https://www.navytimes.com/news/your-navy/2018/06/22/new-navy-parental-leave-policy-gives-new-parents-additional-flexibility/.

8. Department of the Navy, "OPNAV Instruction 6000.1A," February 21, 1989, http://www.operationalmedicine.org/ed2/Instructions/Navy/6000a1.pdf; Department of the Navy, "OPNAV Instruction 6000.1B," March 4, 2003, http://www.operationalmedicine.org/ed2/Instructions/6000.1B.pdf; Department of the Navy, "OPNAV Instruction 6000.1C," June 14, 2007, http://doni.daps.dla.mil/Directives/06000%20Medical%20and%20Dental%20Services/06-00%20General%20Medical%20and%20Dental%20Support%20Services/6000.1C.PDF.

9. This is ironic, given that the new Instructions, OPNAVIST 6001.D state, "Pregnancy and parenthood are natural events that may occur in Service members' lives and can be compatible with successful naval service." Department of the Navy, "OPNAV Instruction 6000.1D," March 12, 2018, https://mccareer.files.wordpress.com/2018/03/opnavinst-6000-1d-navy-guidelines-concerning-pregnancy-and-parenthood.pdf.

10. Eric K. Fanning, "Army Directive 2015-43 (Revised Breastfeeding and Lactation Support)," Department of the Army, November 10, 2015, https://armypubs.army.mil/epubs/DR_pubs/DR_a/pdf/web/ad2015_43.pdf.

11. Department of the Air Force, "Air Force Instruction 44-102," March 17, 2015, 44, https://static.e-publishing.af.mil/production/1/af_sg/publication/afi44-102/afi44-102.pdf.

12. Janet Smithson and Elizabeth H. Stokoe, "Discourses of Work–Life Balance: Negotiating 'Genderblind' Terms in Organizations," *Gender, Work & Organization* 12, no. 2 (2005): 164.

13. Smithson and Stokoe, "Discourses of Work–Life Balance," 157.

14. Sabine Sczesny, Magda Formanowicz, and Franziska Moser, "Can Gender-Fair Language Reduce Gender Stereotyping and Discrimination?," *Frontiers in Psychology* 7, no. 25 (February 2, 2016), https://doi.org/10.3389/fpsyg.2016.00025.

15. Robert L. Wilkie, "Parental Leave for Military Personnel in Connection with the Birth or Adoption of a Child," March 23, 2018, https://localtvwtkr.files.wordpress.com/2018/06/mplp-signed-policy.pdf.

16. Chief of Naval Personnel Public Affairs, "Navy Releases New Parental Leave Program," Navy.Mil, June 21, 2018, http://www.navy.mil/submit/display.asp?story_id=106087.

17. Wilkie, "Parental Leave for Military Personnel," 4.

18. Department of the Navy, "MARADMIN 331/18," June 14, 2018, https://www.marines.mil/News/Messages/MARADMINS/Article/1550376/changes-to-parental-leave-policy/; Undersecretary of Defense,

"NAVADMIN 151/18: Military Parental Leave Program"; Department of the Air Force, "Air Force Instruction 36-3003," August 24, 2020, https://static.e-publishing.af.mil/production/1/af_a1/publication/afi36-3003/afi36-3003.pdf.

19. Amy Barron Smolinski, "Military Parental Leave Program—Not Exactly as Promised," MomsRising.org, November 8, 2018, https://www.momsrising.org/blog/military-parental-leave-program-not-exactly-as-promised

20. Lucinda Joy Peach, "Gender Ideology and the Ethics of Women in Combat," in *It's Our Military Too: Women and the U.S Military*, ed. Judith Stiehm (Philadelphia: Temple University Press, 1996), 171.

21. To read more about the barriers men face when needing or wanting to take family leave, see Amanda Lenhart, Haley Swenson, and Brigid Schulte, "Lifting the Barriers to Paid Family and Medical Leave for Men in the United States," New America, accessed June 23, 2020, http://newamerica.org/better-life-lab/reports/lifting-barriers-paid-family-and-medical-leave-men-united-states/.

22. Nancy Montgomery, "Army Uniform Designed for Women Now for All," *Stars and Stripes*, September 28, 2012, https://www.stripes.com/news/army-uniform-designed-for-women-now-for-all-1.191106.

23. Amme-Marie Slaughter, *Unfinished Business: Women Men Work Family*, reprint ed. (New York: Random House, 2016), 51.

24. Rosa Brooks, "Recline, Don't 'Lean In' (Why I Hate Sheryl Sandberg)," *Washington Post*, February 25, 2014, https://www.washingtonpost.com/blogs/she-the-people/wp/2014/02/25/recline-dont-lean-in-why-i-hate-sheryl-sandberg/.

25. Nikki C. Townsley and Kirsten J. Broadfoot, "Care, Career, and Academe: Heeding the Calls of a New Professoriate," *Women's Studies in Communication* 31, no. 2 (Summer 2008): 137, https://doi.org/10.1080/07491409.2008.10162525.

26. Townsley and Broadfoot, "Care, Career, and Academe," 137.

27. Caitlin Gibson, "The End of Leaning In: How Sheryl Sandberg's Message of Empowerment Fully Unraveled," *Washington Post*, December 20, 2018, https://www.washingtonpost.com/lifestyle/style/the-end-of-lean-in-how-sheryl-sandbergs-message-of-empowerment-fully-unraveled/2018/12/19/9561eb06-fe2e-11e8-862a-b6a6f3ce8199_story.html.

28. Gibson, "The End of Leaning In."

29. Brooks, "Recline, Don't 'Lean In.'"

30. Brooks, "Recline, Don't 'Lean In.'"

31. Department of Defense, *2017 Demographics: Profile of the Military Community*, 2017, http://download.militaryonesource.mil/12038/MOS/Reports/2017-demographics-report.pdf.

32. Department of Defense, *2017 Demographics*, 125.

33. Mark D. Faram, "SECNAV Orders Review of Fitness, Advancement Changes," *Navy Times*, June 12, 2015, https://www.navytimes.com/story/military/careers/2015/06/12/navy-personnel-initiatives-mabus-alnav/71017838/; Ray Mabus, "DoN Talent Management Address to the Brigade of Midshipmen," Annapolis, MD, May 13, 2015, 4, https://news.usni.org/2015/05/15/video-secnav-ray-mabus-speech-on-navy-personnel-changes. Currently, servicewomen comprise about 17 percent of the military according to George M. Reynolds and Amanda Shendruk, "Demographics of the U.S. Military," Council on Foreign Relations, April 24, 2018, https://www.cfr.org/article/demographics-us-military.

34. Department of the Navy, "SECNAV Instruction 1000.10B," January 16, 2019., https://tinyurl.com/SECNAVINST1000.

35. Department of the Navy, "OPNAV Instruction 6000.1C," June 14, 2007, http://doni.daps.dla.mil/Directives/06000%20Medical%20and%20Dental%20Services/06-00%20General%20Medical%20and%20Dental%20Support%20Services/6000.

36. Navy Personnel Command, "Pregnancy and Parenthood," United States Navy, accessed July 18, 2019, https://www.public.navy.mil/bupers-npc/support/21st_Century_Sailor/PregnancyParenthood/Pages/default.aspx.

37. Felice N. Schwartz, "Management Women and the New Facts of Life," *Women in Management Review* 4, no. 5 (May 1989): 74, https://doi.org/10.1108/EUM0000000001789.

38. Schwartz, "Management Women and the New Facts of Life."

39. Slaughter discusses how the "up-or-out" culture is prevalent in most of corporate America, not just in academia or the military. Slaughter, *Unfinished Business*.

Bibliography

Acker, Joan. "Hierarchies, Jobs, Bodies: A Theory of Gendered Organizations." *Gender & Society* 4, no. 2 (June 1, 1990): 139–58. https://doi.org/10.1177/089124390004002002.
Adamczyk, Alicia. "These Are the Companies with the Best Parental Leave Policies." Money, November 4, 2015. http://time.com/money/4098469/paid-parental-leave-google-amazon-apple-facebook/.
Air Force's Personnel Center. "Career Intermission Program." Accessed June 7, 2019. https://www.afpc.af.mil/Career-Management/CIP/.
Alcoff, Linda Martín. "Identities: Modern and Postmodern." In *Identities: Race, Class, Gender, and Nationality*, 1–8. Malden, MA: Blackwell Publishing, 2003.
Alphonse, Lylah. "Military Moms Breastfeeding in Uniform Stir Controversy." Yahoo! Shine, May 12, 2012. http://shine.yahoo.com/parenting/military-moms-breastfeeding-uniform-stir-controversey-214500503.html.
Anderson, Karrin. "Breast of Times, Worst of Times: 'Nursing in Uniform' Photos Draw Fire." Reading the Pictures, May 31, 2012, https://www.readingthepictures.org/2012/05/breast-of-times-worst-of-times-nursing-in-uniform-photos-draw-fire/.

Ansel, Bridget. "Is the Cost of Childcare Driving Women out of the U.S. Workforce?" *Equitable Growth*, November 29, 2016. https://equitablegrowth.org/is-the-cost-of-childcare-driving-women-out-of-the-u-s-workforce/.

Ashcraft, Karen Lee. "Managing Maternity Leave: A Qualitative Analysis of Temporary Executive Succession." *Administrative Science Quarterly* 44 (1999): 240–80.

Baldor, Lolita C. "US Navy Triples Paid Maternity Leave in Effort to Attract Women." Military.com, July 3, 2015. http://www.military.com/daily-news/2015/07/03/us-navy-triple-paid-maternity-leave-in-effort-to-attract-women.html.

Banks, Nina. "Black Women's Labor Market History Reveals Deep-Seated Race and Gender Discrimination." Economic Policy Institute, February 19, 2019. https://www.epi.org/blog/black-womens-labor-market-history-reveals-deep-seated-race-and-gender-discrimination/.

Barrett, Frank J. "The Organizational Construction of Hegemonic Masculinity: The Case of the US Navy." *Gender, Work & Organization* 3, no. 3 (1996): 129–42.

Bassett, Laura. "Military Abortion Amendment Is Included in Final Defense Bill." *Huffington Post*, December 18, 2012. http://www.huffingtonpost.com/2012/12/18/military-abortion-amendment_n_2324969.html.

Beauvoir, Simone de. *The Second Sex*. New York: Vintage, 1989.

Bemis, Bethanee. "Pregnant in Uniform." National Museum of American History, September 26, 2011. https://americanhistory.si.edu/blog/2011/09/pregnant-in-uniform.html.

Biank, Tanya. *Undaunted: The Real Story of America's Servicewomen in Today's Military*. New York: Penguin, 2014.

Biggs, R. Lee, Brad H. Douglas, Amy L. O'Boyle, and Thomas S. Rieg. "The Impact of Pregnancy on the Individual and Military Organization: A Postpartum Active Duty Survey." *Military Medicine* 174, no. 1 (2009): 61–75.

Blair-Loy, Mary. "Cultural Constructions of Family Schemas: The Case of Women Finance Executives." *Gender & Society* 15, no. 5 (2001): 687–709.

Bologna, Caroline. "Air Force Mom Breastfeeding in Uniform Is a Stunning Look at Military Motherhood." *HuffPost*, March 12, 2015. https://www.huffpost.com/entry/jonea-cunico-military-breastfeed_n_6856762.

———. "7 Powerful Photos of Military Moms Breastfeeding in Uniform." *HuffPost*, May 12, 2016. https://www.huffpost.com/entry/7-powerful-photos-of-military-moms-breastfeeding-in-uniform_n_5730aa94e4b0bc9cb0475f14.

Borda, Jennifer. "Lean In or Leave before You Leave?: False Dichotomies of Choice and Blame in Public Debates about Working Motherhood." In *The Mother Blame-Game*, edited by Vanessa Reimer and Sarah Sahagian, 219–36. Toronto, ON: Demeter Press, 2005.

Bradner, Eric. "U.S. Military Opens Combat Positions to Women." CNN, December 3, 2015. https://www.cnn.com/2015/12/03/politics/u-s-military-women-combat-positions/index.html.

Braidotti, Rosi. "Mothers, Monsters, and Machines." In *Writing on the Body: Female Embodiment and Feminist Theory*, edited by Katie Conboy, Nadia Medina, and Sarah Stanbury, 59–79. New York: Columbia University Press, 1997.

Britt, Elizabeth C. *Conceiving Normalcy: Rhetoric, Law, and the Double Binds of Infertility*. Tuscaloosa: University of Alabama Press, 2001.

———. *Reimagining Advocacy: Rhetorical Education in the Legal Clinic*. University Park, Pennsylvania: Penn State University Press, 2018.

Brooks, Rosa. "Recline, Don't 'Lean In' (Why I Hate Sheryl Sandberg)." *Washington Post*, February 25, 2014. https://www.washingtonpost.com/blogs/she-the-people/wp/2014/02/25/recline-dont-lean-in-why-i-hate-sheryl-sandberg/.

Brown, Melissa T. *Enlisting Masculinity: The Construction of Gender in US Military Recruiting Advertising during the All-Volunteer Force*. New York: Oxford University Press, 2012.

Buchanan, Lindal. *Rhetorics of Motherhood*. Carbondale: Southern Illinois University Press, 2013.

Bullis, Connie, and Karen Rohrbauck Stout. "Organizational Socialization: A Feminist Standpoint Approach." In *Rethinking Organizational and Managerial Communication from Feminist Perspectives*, edited by Patrice M. Buzzanell. Thousand Oaks, CA: Sage, 2000.

Burke, Carol. "Military Folk Culture." In *Beyond Zero Tolerance: Discrimination in Military Culture*, edited by Mary Fainsod Katzenstein and Judith Reppy, 53–63. Lanham, MD: Rowman & Littlefield Publishers, 1999.

Bushatz, Amy. "Breastfeeding Policy Will Help Army Retain Female Soldiers: Lawmaker." Military.Com, December 17, 2015. http://www.military.com/daily-news/2015/12/17/breastfeeding-policy-help-army-retain-female-soldiers-lawmaker.html.

———. "Pentagon Sets Maternity Leave at 12 Weeks for All Services." Military.com, January 28, 2016. http://www.military.com/daily-news/2016/01/28/maternity-leave-slashed-for-sailors-marines.html.

Buzzanell, Patrice M. "Reframing the Glass Ceiling as a Socially Constructed Process: Implications for Understanding and Change." *Communication Monographs* 62 (1995): 327–54.

Buzzanell, Patrice M., and Laura L. Ellingson. "Contesting Narratives of Workplace Maternity." In *Narratives, Health, and Healing: Communication Theory, Research, and Practice*, edited by Lynn M. Harter, Phyllis M. Japp, and Christina S. Beck, 277–94. Mahwah, NJ: Lawrence Erlbaum, 2005.

Buzzanell, Patrice M., and Meina Liu. "It's 'Give and Take': Maternity Leave as a Conflict Management Process." *Human Relations* 60, no. 3 (March 1, 2007): 463–95. https://doi.org/10.1177/0018726707076688.

———. "Struggling with Maternity Leave Policies and Practices: A Poststructuralist Feminist Analysis of Gendered Organizing." *Journal of Applied Communication Research* 33, no. 1 (February 2005): 1–25. https://doi.org/10.1080/0090988042000318495.

Buzzanell, Patrice M., Rebecca Meisenbach, Robyn Remke, Meina Liu, Venessa Bowers, and Cindy Conn. "The Good *Working* Mother: Managerial Women's Sensemaking and Feelings about Work–Family Issues." *Communication Studies* 56, no. 3 (January 2005): 261–85. https://doi.org/10.1080/10510970500181389.

Carroll, Ginny, and Carol Barkalow. "Women Have What It Takes." *Newsweek*, August 5, 1991.

Charland, Maurice. "Constitutive Rhetoric: The Case of the Peuple Québécois." *Quarterly Journal of Speech* 73, no. 2 (1987): 133–50.

Cheney, George, and Daniel J. Lair. "Theorizing about Rhetoric and Organizations." In *Engaging Organizational Communication Theory and Research: Multiple Perspectives*, edited by Steve May and Dennis K. Mumby, 55–84. Thousand Oaks, CA: Sage, 2005. http://dx.doi.org/10.4135/9781452204536.n4.

Chief of Naval Personnel Public Affairs. "Navy Releases New Parental Leave Program." Navy.Mil, June 21, 2018. http://www.navy.mil/submit/display.asp?story_id=106087.

Collett, Jessica L. "What Kind of Mother Am I?: Impression Management and the Social Construction of Motherhood." *Symbolic Interaction* 28, no. 3 (August 2005): 327–47. https://doi.org/10.1525/si.2005.28.3.327.

Comack, Elizabeth, and Tracey Peter. "How the Criminal Justice System Responds to Sexual Assault Survivors: The Slippage between 'Responsibilization' and 'Blaming the Victim.'" *Canadian Journal of Women and the Law* 17, no. 2 (2005): 283–309. https://doi.org/10.1353/jwl.2007.0002.

Connell, R. W. *Masculinities*. 2nd ed. Berkeley: University of California Press, 2005.

———. "Masculinity, Violence, and War." In *War/Masculinity*, edited by Paul Patton and Ross Poole. Sydney, Australia: Intervention, 1985.

Copp, Tara. "Carter: '1 or 2' Years More in Rank with Proposed 'Up or Out' Policy Changes." *Stars and Stripes*, June 23, 2016. https://www.stripes.com/news/carter-1-or-2-years-more-in-rank-with-proposed-up-or-out-policy-changes-1.415892#.WXDHCIqQyRt.

Crawford v. Cushman, 531 Federal Reporter 1114 (United States Court of Appeals Second Circuit 1976).

DeLuca, Kevin Michael. *Image Politics the New Rhetoric of Environmental Activism*. Mahwah, NJ: Lawrence Erlbaum, 1999.

D'Enbeau, Suzy, and Patrice M. Buzzanell. "Efficiencies of Pregnancy Management." In *Culture of Efficiency: Technology in Everyday Life*, edited by Sharon Kleinman, 3–19. New York: Peter Lang, 2009.

Department of Defense. *2017 Demographics: Profile of the Military Community*. 2017. http://download.militaryonesource.mil/12038/MOS/Reports/2017-demographics-report.pdf.

Department of the Air Force. "Air Force Instruction 36-3003. AFGM2018-01." June 6, 2018. https://static.e-publishing.af.mil/production/1/af_a1/publication/afi36-3003/afi36-3003.pdf.

———. "Air Force Instruction 44-102," March 17, 2015, 44. http://static.e-publishing.af.mil/production/1/af_sg/publication/afi44-102/afi44-102.pdf.

Department of the Navy. "MARADMIN 331/18." June 14, 2018. https://www.marines.mil/News/Messages/MARADMINS/Article/1550376/changes-to-parental-leave-policy/.

———. "NAVADMIN 151/18." June 2018. http://www.public.navy.mil/bupers-npc/reference/messages/Documents/NAVADMINS/NAV2018/NAV18151.txt.

———. "OPNAV Instruction 6000.1A." February 21, 1989. http://www.operationalmedicine.org/ed2/Instructions/Navy/6000a1.pdf.

———. "OPNAV Instruction 6000.1B." March 4, 2003. http://www.operationalmedicine.org/ed2/Instructions/6000.1B.pdf.

———. "OPNAV Instruction 6000.1C." June 14, 2007. http://doni.daps.dla.mil/Directives/06000%20Medical%20and%20Dental%20Services/06-00%20General%20Medical%20and%20Dental%20Support%20Services/6000.1C.PDF.

———. "OPNAV Instruction 6000.1D." March 12, 2018. https://mccareer.files.wordpress.com/2018/03/opnavinst-6000-1d-navy-guidelines-concerning-pregnancy-and-parenthood.pdf.

———. OPNAV (N130). "MILPERSMAN 1050-435: Maternity Leave." U.S. Navy, November 18, 2016. https://www.public.navy.mil/bupers-npc/reference/milpersman/1000/1000General/Documents/1050-435.pdf.

———. "SECNAV Instruction 1000.10B," January 16, 2019. https://tinyurl.com/SECNAVINST1000.

Douglas, Susan, and Meredith Michaels. *The Mommy Myth: The Idealization of Motherhood and How It Has Undermined All Women*. New York: Free Press, 2004.

Dubbert, Joe. *Man's Place: Masculinity in Transition*. Englewood Cliffs, NJ: Prentice Hall, 1979.

Dubriwny, Tasha N. "Consciousness-Raising as Collective Rhetoric: The Articulation of Experience in the Redstockings' Abortion Speak-Out of 1969." *Quarterly Journal of Speech* 91, no. 4 (November 2005): 395–422. https://doi.org/10.1080/00335630500488275.

Duke, M. R., and G. M. Ames. "Challenges of Contraceptive Use and Pregnancy Prevention among Women in the U.S. Navy." *Qualitative Health Research* 18, no. 2 (February 1, 2008): 244–53. https://doi.org/10.1177/1049732307312305.

Dunivan, Karen O. "Military Culture: Change and Continuity." *Armed Forces & Society* 20, no. 4 (1994): 531–47.

Elshtain, Jean Bethke. *Women and War* (with a new epilogue). Chicago: University of Chicago Press, 1995.

Enloe, Cynthia. "Beyond Steve Canyon and Rambo: Feminist Histories of Militarized Masculinity." In *Militarization of Western World*, edited by John Gillis, 119–40. New Brunswick, NJ: Rutgers University Press, 1989.

———. *Does Khaki Become You?: The Militarisation of Women's Lives*. London: Pluto Press Limited, 1983.

———. *Globalization and Militarism: Feminists Make the Link*. Lanham, MD: Rowman & Littlefield, 2007.

———. *Maneuvers: The International Politics of Militarizing Women's Lives*. Berkeley: University of California Press, 2000.

Evans, Mary Ann, and Leora Rosen. "Pregnancy Planning and the Impact on Work Climate, Psychological Well-Being, and Work Effort in the Military." *Journal of Occupational Health Psychology* 2, no. 4 (1997): 353.

Eyer, Diane. *Motherguilt: How Our Culture Blames Mothers for What's Wrong with Society*. New York: Random House, 1996.

Fanning, Eric K. "Army Directive 2015-43 (Revised Breastfeeding and Lactation Support)." Department of the Army, November 10, 2015 .https://armypubs.army.mil/epubs/DR_pubs/DR_a/pdf/web/ad2015_43.pdf.

Faram, Mark D. "SECNAV Orders Review of Fitness, Advancement Changes." *Navy Times*, June 12, 2015. https://www.navytimes.com/story/military/careers/2015/06/12/navy-personnel-initiatives-mabus-alnav/71017838/.

——. "Sweeping Uniform Changes Emphasize Gender Neutrality." *Navy Times*, August 22, 2017. https://www.navytimes.com/news/your-navy/2015/10/09/sweeping-uniform-changes-emphasize-gender-neutrality/.

Fitzgerald, April S., Rita L. Duboyce, Joan B. Ritter, Deborah J. Omori, Barbara A. Cooper, and Patrick G. O'Malley. "A Primer on the Unique Challenges of Female Soldiers' Reproductive Issues in a War-Ready Culture." *Military Medicine* 178, no. 5 (May 2013): 511–16. https://doi.org/10.7205/MILMED-D-12-00384.

Fixmer-Oraiz, Natalie. "Contemplating Homeland Maternity." *Women's Studies in Communication* 38, no. 2 (April 3, 2015): 129–34. https://doi.org/10.1080/07491409.2015.1034630.

——. *Homeland Maternity: US Security Culture and the New Reproductive Regime*. Urbana: University of Illinois Press, 2019.

Flores vs. Secretary of Defense, 355 Federal Supplement 93 (United States District Court for the Northern District of Florida, Pensacola Division, 1973).

Foss, Sonja K. *Rhetorical Criticism: Exploration and Practice*. 5th edition. Long Grove, IL: Waveland Press, Inc., 2017.

Foucault, Michel. *Discipline and Punish: The Birth of the Prison*. 2nd ed. New York: Vintage, 1995.

——. *The History of Sexuality, Vol. 1: An Introduction*. Translated by Robert Hurley. New York: Vintage, 1976.

Frost, Nollaig, and Frauke Elichaoff. "Feminist Postmodernism, Poststructuralism, and Critical Theory." In *Feminist Research Practice: A*

Primer, edited by Sharlene Hesse-Biber, 2nd ed., 42–72. Los Angeles, CA: Sage, 2014.

Gaines, Atwood D., and Robbie Davis-Floyd. "Biomedicine." In *Encyclopedia of Medical Anthropology: Health and Illness in the World's Cultures*, edited by Carol R. Ember and Melvin Ember, vol. 1. New York: Kluwer Academic/Plenum Publishers, 2004.

Gaonkar, Dilip Parameshwar. "Performing with Fragments: Reflections on Critical Rhetoric." *Argument and the Postmodern Challenge: Proceedings from the Eighth SCA/AFA Conference on Argumentation*, 1993, 149–55.

Gerrard, Meg, Frederick X. Gibbons, and Teddy D. Warner. "Effects of Reviewing Risk-Relevant Behavior on Perceived Vulnerability among Women Marines." *Health Psychology* 10, no. 3 (1991): 173.

Gibson, Caitlin. "The End of Leaning In: How Sheryl Sandberg's Message of Empowerment Fully Unraveled." *Washington Post*, December 20, 2018. https://www.washingtonpost.com/lifestyle/style/the-end-of-lean-in-how-sheryl-sandbergs-message-of-empowerment-fully-unraveled/2018/12/19/9561eb06-fe2e-11e8-862a-b6a6f3ce8199_story.html.

Gill, Rosalind. "Postfeminist Media Culture: Elements of a Sensibility." *European Journal of Cultural Studies* 10, no. 2 (2007): 147–66.

Goffman, Erving. *Stigma: Notes on the Management of Spoiled Identity*. New York: Simon and Schuster, 1963.

Goldstein, Joshua S. *War and Gender: How Gender Shapes the War System and Vice Versa*. Cambridge: Cambridge University Press, 2001.

Gray, G. C. "The Responsibilization Strategy of Health and Safety: Neo-Liberalism and the Reconfiguration of Individual Responsibility for Risk." *British Journal of Criminology* 49, no. 3 (January 6, 2009): 326–42. https://doi.org/10.1093/bjc/azp004.

Greenberg, Jon. "Yes, the United States Is the Only Industrialized Nation without Paid Family Leave." *PolitiFact*, July 25, 2016. https://www.politifact.com/truth-o-meter/statements/2016/jul/25/kirsten-gillibrand/yes-us-only-industrialized-nation-without-paid-fam/.

Grinberg, Emanuella. "Soldiers in Camo Breastfeed in Photo." CNN, September 15, 2015. https://www.cnn.com/2015/09/13/living/breastfeeding-soldiers-uniform-feat/index.html.

Grindlay, Kate. "A Guide to Birth Control When You're in the Military." *Bedsider*, November 8, 2016. https://www.bedsider.org/features/967-a-guide-to-birth-control-when-you-re-in-the-military.

Grindlay, Kate, and Daniel Grossman. "Contraception Access and Use among U.S. Servicewomen during Deployment." *Contraception* 87, no. 2 (2013): 162–69. https://doi.org/10.1016/j.contraception.2012.09.019.

———. "Unintended Pregnancy among Active-Duty Women in the United States Military, 2008." *Obstetrics & Gynecology* 121, no. 2, PART 1 (2013): 241–46.

Guenter-Schlesinger, Sue. "Persistence of Sexual Harassment: The Impact of Military Culture on Policy Implementation." In *Beyond Zero Tolerance: Discrimination in Military Culture*, edited by Mary Fainsod Katzenstein and Judith Reppy, 195–212. Lanham, MD: Rowman & Littlefield, 1999.

Gupta, Alisha Haridasani. "Why Some Women Call This Recession a 'Shesession.'" *New York Times*, May 9, 2020. https://www.nytimes.com/2020/05/09/us/unemployment-coronavirus-women.html.

Gutmann, Stephanie. "Sex and the Soldier." *The New Republic*, February 24, 1997.

Hannah-Moffat, Kelly. *Punishment in Disguise: Penal Governance and Federal Imprisonment of Women in Canada*. Toronto: University of Toronto Press, 2001.

Haraway, Donna. *Simians, Cyborgs, and Women: The Reinvention of Nature*. New York: Routledge, 1991.

———. "Situated Knowledges: The Science Question in Feminism and the Privilege of Partial Perspectives." *Feminist Studies* 14, no. 3 (1988): 575–99.

Hasian, Marouf, Jr. "The 'Hysterical' Emily Hobhouse and Boer War Concentration Camp Controversy." *Western Journal of Communication* 67, no. 2 (Spring 2003): 138–63. https://doi.org/10.1080/10570310309374764.

Hayden, Sara, and D. Lynn O'Brien Hallstein, eds. *Contemplating Maternity in an Era of Choice: Explorations into Discourses of Reproduction*. Lanham, MD: Lexington Books, 2010.

———. "Introduction." In *Contemplating Maternity in an Era of Choice: Explorations into Discourses of Reproduction*, edited by Sara Hayden and D. Lynn O'Brien Hallstein, xiii–xxxix. Lanham, MD: Lexington Books, 2010.

Hays, Sharon. *The Cultural Contradictions of Motherhood*. New Haven, CT: Yale University Press, 1996.

Heisler, Jennifer M., and Jennifer Butler Ellis. "Motherhood and the Construction of 'Mommy Identity': Messages about Motherhood and Face Negotiation." *Communication Quarterly* 56, no. 4 (November 19, 2008): 445–67. https://doi.org/10.1080/01463370802448246.

Heitmann, Ryan J., Alison L. Batig, Gary Levy, Jonathan Novotney, Calvin Grubbs, Timothy S. Batig, Joseph M. Gobern, Eileen Hemman, Alicia Y. Christy, and Micah J. Hill. "Unintended Pregnancy in the Military Health Care System: Who Is Really at Risk?" *Military Medicine* 181, no. 10 (October 2016): 1370–74. https://doi.org/10.7205/MILMED-D-16-00003.

Hesse-Biber, Sharlene. "A Re-Invitation of Feminist Research." In *Feminist Research Practice: A Primer*, edited by Sharlene Hesse-Biber, 2nd ed., 1–13. Los Angeles, CA: Sage, 2014.

Higate, Paul. *Military Masculinities: Identity and the State*. Westport, CT: Praeger, 2003.

Hodnet, Ellen D. "Continuity of Caregivers for Care during Pregnancy and Childbirth." *Cochrane Database of Systematic Reviews*, no. 1 (2000). https://doi.org/10.1002/14651858.CD000062.

Holm, Jeanne. *Women in the Military: An Unfinished Revolution*. New York: Presidio Press, 1993.

Holt, Kelsey, Kate Grindlay, Madeline Taskier, and Daniel Grossman. "Unintended Pregnancy and Contraceptive Use among Women in the US Military: A Systematic Literature Review." *Military Medicine* 176, no. 9 (2011): 1056–64.

Ivie, Robert L. "Productive Criticism Then and Now." *American Communication Journal* 4, no. 3 (2001). http://ac-journal.org/journal/vol4/iss3/special/ivie.pdf.

Jacobson, Janet C., and Jeffrey T. Jensen. "A Policy of Discrimination: Reproductive Health Care in the Military." *Women's Health Issues* 21, no. 4 (July 2011): 255–58. https://doi.org/10.1016/j.whi.2011.03.008.

Jade Beall Photography's Facebook Page. "Jonea Cunico," March 3, 2015. https://www.facebook.com/JadeBeallPhotography/photos/a.1930387 24076942.48997.193035750743906/831187540262054/?type=1.

Jarvis, Christina S. *The Male Body at War: American Masculinity during World War II*. DeKalb: Northern Illinois University Press, 2010.

Jasinski, James. *Sourcebook on Rhetoric: Key Concepts in Contemporary Rhetorical Studies*. Thousand Oaks, CA: Sage, 2001. https://doi.org/10.4135/9781452233222.

Jensen, Robin E. *Infertility: Tracing the History of a Transformative Term*. University Park: Pennsylvania State University Press, 2016.

Johnson, Paula A., Sheila E. Widnall, and Frazier F. Benya, eds. *Sexual Harassment of Women: Climate, Culture, and Consequences in Academic Sciences, Engineering, and Medicine*. Washington, DC: The National Academies Press, 2018.

Johnston, Deirdre D., and Debra H. Swanson. "Cognitive Acrobatics in the Construction of Worker–Mother Identity." *Sex Roles* 57, nos. 5–6 (August 21, 2007): 447–59. https://doi.org/10.1007/s11199-007-9267-4.

Jordan, Bryant. "US Navy Triples Maternity Leave to 18 Weeks for Sailors and Marines." *Military.Com*, August 6, 2015. http://www.military.com/daily-news/2015/08/06/us-navy-triples-maternity-leave-to-18-weeks-for-sailors-marines.html.

Jowers, Karen. "More Bases Offering Extended Child Care Hours." *Military Times*, October 6, 2017. https://www.militarytimes.com/pay-benefits/2017/10/06/more-bases-offering-extended-child-care-hours/.

Kamarck, Kristy N. "Women in Combat: Issues for Congress." Congressional Research Service, December 3, 2015. https://fas.org/sgp/crs/natsec/R42075.pdf.

Kaplan, Fred. "The U.S. Army Lowers Recruitment Standards . . . Again." *Slate*, January 24, 2008. http://www.slate.com/articles/news_and_politics/war_stories/2008/01/dumb_and_dumber.html.

Katzenstein, Mary Fainsod, and Judith Reppy, eds. *Beyond Zero Tolerance: Discrimination in Military Culture*. Lanham, MD: Rowman & Littlefield Publishers, 1999.

Kids Count Data Center. "Children under Age 6 with All Available Parents in the Labor Force." The Annie E. Casey Foundation Kids Count Data Center, October 2018. https://datacenter.kidscount.org/data/Tables/5057-children-under-age-6-with-all-available-parents-in-the-labor-force.

Kimmel, Michael S. "Masculinity as Homophobia." In *The Social Construction of Difference and Inequality*, edited by T. E. Ore, 2nd ed., 119–36. Boston: McGraw-Hill, 2003.

Kitroeff, Natalie. "Why Are So Many Women Dropping Out of the Workforce?" *Los Angeles Times*, May 28, 2017. http://www.latimes.com/business/la-fi-women-dropping-out-20170522-story.html.

Ko, Jean Y., Karilynn M. Rockhill, Van T. Tong, Brian Morrow, and Sherry L. Farr. "Trends in Postpartum Depressive Symptoms—27 States, 2004, 2008, and 2012." *Morbidity and Mortality Weekly Report* 66, no. 6 (2017): 153–58. https://doi.org/10.15585/mmwr.mm6606a1.

Koerber, Amy. *Breast or Bottle?: Contemporary Controversies in Infant-Feeding Policy and Practice*. Columbia: University of South Carolina Press, 2013.

———. *From Hysteria to Hormones: A Rhetorical History*. University Park: Pennsylvania State University Press, 2018.

Kornfield, Sarah. "Pregnant Discourse: 'Having It All' While Domestic and Potentially Disabled." *Women's Studies in Communication* 37, no. 2 (May 4, 2014): 181–201. https://doi.org/10.1080/07491409.2014.911233.

Kube, Courtney, and Jim Miklaszewski. "Military to Announce Changes to Maternity Leave Policy." NBC News, January 28, 2016. http://www.nbcnews.com/news/us-news/military-announce-changes-maternity-leave-policy-n506006.

Kwolek, Laurie A., Cristobal S. Berry-Caban, and Sean F. Thomas. "Pregnant Soldiers' Participation in Physical Training: A Descriptive Study." *Military Medicine* 176, no. 8 (2011): 926–31.

Lenhart, Amanda, Haley Swenson, and Brigid Schulte. "Lifting the Barriers to Paid Family and Medical Leave for Men in the United States." New America. Accessed June 23, 2020. http://newamerica.org/better-life-lab/reports/lifting-barriers-paid-family-and-medical-leave-men-united-states/.

Lerner, Sharon. "The Real War on Families: Why the U.S. Needs Paid Leave Now." *In These Times*, August 18, 2015. http://inthesetimes.com/article/18151/the-real-war-on-families.

Long, Heather. "Did Donald Trump Endorse Paid FAMILY Leave?" CNNMoney, March 6, 2017. https://money.cnn.com/2017/03/06/news/economy/donald-trump-paid-family-leave/index.html.

Losey, Stephen. "New Air Force Policy Gives New Mothers 12 Months to Decide If They Want to Stay in Uniform." *Air Force Times*, April 29, 2017. https://www.airforcetimes.com/news/your-air-force/2017/04/29/new-air-force-policy-gives-new-mothers-12-months-to-decide-if-they-want-to-stay-in-uniform/.

Ludden, Jennifer. "FMLA Not Really Working for Many Employees." NPR, February 5, 2013. https://www.npr.org/2013/02/05/171078451/fmla-not-really-working-for-many-employees.

Lundquist, Jennifer Hickes, and Herbert L. Smith. "Family Formation among Women in the US Military: Evidence from the NLSY." *Journal of Marriage and Family* 67, no. 1 (2005): 1–13.

Mabus, Ray. "DoN Talent Management Address to the Brigade of Midshipmen." Annapolis, MD, May 13, 2015. https://news.usni.org/2015/05/15/video-secnav-ray-mabus-speech-on-navy-personnel-changes.
———. "Video: SECNAV Ray Mabus Speech on Navy Personnel Changes." *USNI News* (blog), May 15, 2015. https://news.usni.org/2015/05/15/video-secnav-ray-mabus-speech-on-navy-personnel-changes.
Machung, Anne. "Talking Career, Thinking Job: Gender Differences in Career and Family Expectations of Berkeley Seniors." *Feminist Studies* 15, no. 1 (1989): 35. https://doi.org/10.2307/3177817.
Mack, Ashley N. "Disciplining Mommy: Rhetorics of Reproduction in Contemporary Maternity Culture." The University of Texas at Austin, 2013. http://repositories.lib.utexas.edu/bitstream/ handle/2152/21299/MACK-DISSERTATION-2013.pdf?sequence=1.
MacKinnon, Catherine A. "Difference and Dominance: On Sex Discrimination." In *Feminism Unmodified: Discourses on Life and Law*, 32–45. Cambridge, MA: Harvard University Press, 1987.
Mackintosh, Virginia H., Miriam Liss, and Holly H. Schiffrin. "Using a Quantitative Measure to Explore Intensive Mothering Ideology." In *Intensive Mothering: The Cultural Contradictions of Modern Motherhood*, edited by Linda Rose Ennis, 142–59. Bradford, ON: Demeter Press, 2014.
Mahadevan, Alex. "Women Are Leaving the Workforce at a Staggering Rate—Here's Why." *The Penny Hoarder*, August 23, 2017. http://www.thepennyhoarder.com/make-money/shrinking-number-of-women-in-the-workforce/.
Martin, Joanne. "Deconstructing Organizational Taboos: The Suppression of Gender Conflict in Organizations." *Organization Science* 1, no. 4 (1990). http://www.jstor.org/stable/pdf/2634968.pdf.
Maucione, Scott. "Why Are So Few Troops Signing Up for One of DoD's Most Flexible Personnel Pilot Programs?" *Federal News Network*, April 3, 2018. https://federalnewsnetwork.com/defense-main/2018/04/taking-a-break-why-one-of-dods-flagship-personnel-programs-is-struggling/.
Mayo Clinic Staff. "High-Risk Pregnancy: Know What to Expect." Mayo Clinic, February 21, 2018. http://www.mayoclinic.org/healthy-lifestyle/pregnancy-week-by-week/in-depth/high-risk-pregnancy/art-20047012.
McCarver, Virginia. "The Rhetoric of Choice and 21st-Century Feminism: Online Conversations about Work, Family, and Sarah Palin." *Women's*

Studies in Communication 34, no. 1 (May 5, 2011): 20–41. https://doi.org/10.1080/07491409.2011.566532.

McFarlane, Megan D. "Breastfeeding as Subversive: Mothers, Mammaries, and the Military." *International Feminist Journal of Politics*, January 29, 2014, 1–18. https://doi.org/10.1080/14616742.2013.849967.

———. "Circuits of Discipline: Intensified Responsibilization and the Double Bind of Pregnancy in the U.S. Military." *Women's Studies in Communication* 41, no. 1 (January 2, 2018): 22–41. https://doi.org/10.1080/07491409.2017.1419525.

———. "U.S. Military Policy and the Discursive Construction of Servicewomen's Bodies." ProQuest Dissertations Publishing, 2015.

McGee, Michael Calvin. "Text, Context, and the Fragmentation of Contemporary Culture." *Western Journal of Speech Communication* 54, no. Summer (1990): 274–89.

McKeon, Howard P. "Buck." National Defense Authorization Act for Fiscal Year 2013, Pub. L. No. H.R.4310.EAS (2012). http://thomas.loc.gov/cgi-bin/query/D?c112:6:./temp/~c112P3QZ32::

McKerrow, Raymie E. "Critical Rhetoric: Theory and Praxis." *Communication Monographs* 56 (June 1989): 91–111.

Meedya, Shahla, Kathleen Fahy, and Ashley Kable. "Factors That Positively Influence Breastfeeding Duration to 6 Months: A Literature Review." *Women and Birth* 23, no. 4 (December 1, 2010): 135–45. https://doi.org/10.1016/j.wombi.2010.02.002.

Meisenbach, Rebecca J., Robyn V. Remke, Patrice Buzzanell, and Meina Liu. "'They Allowed': Pentadic Mapping of Women's Maternity Leave Discourse as Organizational Rhetoric." *Communication Monographs* 75, no. 1 (March 1, 2008): 1–24. https://doi.org/10.1080/03637750801952727.

Middleton, Michael, Aaron Hess, Danielle Endres, and Samantha Senda-Cook. *Participatory Critical Rhetoric: Theoretical and Methodological Foundations for Studying Rhetoric In Situ*. Lanham, MD: Lexington, 2017.

Middleton, Michael, Samantha Senda-Cook, and Danielle Endres. "Articulating Rhetorical Field Methods: Challenges and Tensions." *Western Journal of Communication* 75, no. 4 (July 2011): 386–406. https://doi.org/10.1080/10570314.2011.586969.

Mom2Momglobal, Breastfeeding in Combat Boots. "Military Policies." Accessed June 6, 2019. https://www.mom2momglobal.org/breastfeeding-in-combat-boots.

Montgomery, Nancy. "Army Uniform Designed for Women Now for All." *Stars and Stripes*, September 28, 2012. https://www.stripes.com/news/army-uniform-designed-for-women-now-for-all-1.191106.

Morgan, David H. "Theater of War: Combat, the Military, and Masculinities." In *Theorizing Masculinities*, edited by Harry Brod and Michael Kaufman, 165–82. Thousand Oaks: SAGE Publications, 1994.

Morison, Tracy, Catriona Macleod, Ingrid Lynch, Magda Mijas, and Seemanthini Tumkur Shivakumar. "Stigma Resistance in Online Childfree Communities: The Limitations of Choice Rhetoric." *Psychology of Women Quarterly* 40, no. 2 (June 2016): 184–98. https://doi.org/10.1177/0361684315603657.

Morning Edition. "Navy, Marine Corps Now Offer 18 Weeks of Maternity Leave." NPR, July 8, 2015. http://www.npr.org/2015/07/08/421083589/navy-marine-corps-now-offer-18-weeks-of-maternity-leave.

Morris, Madeline. "In War and Peace: Incidence and Implications of Rape by Military Personnel." In *Beyond Zero Tolerance: Discrimination in Military Culture*, edited by Mary Fainsod Katzenstein and Judith Reppy, 163–94. Lanham, MD: Rowman & Littlefield Publishers, 1999.

Moye, Jay. "Paid Leave for All Parents: Millennial Employees Drive Coke's New Parental Benefits Policy." The Coca-Cola Company, April 11, 2016. https://www.coca-colacompany.com/stories/paid-leave-for-all-parents--millennial-employees-drive-cokes-new/.

Murnane, Linda Strite. "Legal Impediments to Service: Women in the Military and the Rule of Law." *Duke Journal Gender Law & Policy* 14 (2007): 1061–96.

Murphy, Alexandra G. "The Dialectical Gaze: Exploring the Subject-Object Tension in the Performances of Women Who Strip." *Journal of Contemporary Ethnography* 32, no. 3 (June 1, 2003): 305–35. https://doi.org/10.1177/0891241603032003003.

Myers, Meghann. "Navy Rolls Back Maternity Leave from 18 to 12 Weeks." *Navy Times*, February 25, 2015. https://www.navytimes.com/story/military/2016/02/25/navy-rolls-back-maternity-leave-18-12-weeks/80939818/.

———. "Navy Triples Maternity Leave for Sailors, Starting Now." *Navy Times*, August 5, 2015. https://www.navytimes.com/story/military/2015/08/05/navy-triples-maternity-leave-sailors-starting-now/31168645/.

Nash, Noah. "New Navy Parental Leave Policy Gives New Parents Additional Flexibility." *Navy Times*, June 22, 2018. https://www.navytimes

.com/news/your-navy/2018/06/22/new-navy-parental-leave-policy
-gives-new-parents-additional-flexibility/.

Naval Physical Readiness Program. "Guide 8: Managing Physical Fitness Assessment Records for Pregnant Servicewomen." U.S. Navy, 2016. http://www.public.navy.mil/bupers-npc/support/21st_Century_Sailor/physical/Documents/Guide%208-%20Managing%20PFA%20Records%20for%20Pregnant%20Service%20Women%202016%20(F).pdf.

Navy Office of Women's Policy. "Women's Policy." Department of the Navy. Accessed February 27, 2014. http://www.public.navy.mil/bupers-npc/organization/bupers/WomensPolicy/Documents/Women%27s%20Policy%20Handout.pdf.

Navy Personnel Command. "Pregnancy and Parenthood." United States Navy. Accessed July 18, 2019. https://www.public.navy.mil/bupers-npc/support/21st_Century_Sailor/PregnancyParenthood/Pages/default.aspx.

———. "Pregnancy FAQs." January 18, 2017. http://www.public.navy.mil/bupers-npc/organization/bupers/WomensPolicy/Pages/FAQs-Women'sPolicy.aspx.

Nemo, Leslie. "The Challenge of Accessing Birth Control in the Military." *Atlantic*, February 23, 2017. https://www.theatlantic.com/health/archive/2017/02/military-women-birth-control/517452/.

O'Brien Hallstein, D. Lynn. "Introduction to Mothering Rhetorics." *Women's Studies in Communication* 40, no. 1 (2017): 1–10. http://dx.doi.org/10.1080/07491409.2017.1280326.

———. "Public Choices, Private Control: How Mediated Mom Labels Work Rhetorically to Dismantle the Politics of Choice and White Second Wave Feminist Successes." In *Contemplating Maternity in an Era of Choice: Explorations into Discourses of Reproduction*, edited by Sara Hayden and D. Lynn O'Brien Hallstein, 5–26. Lanham, MD: Lexington Books, 2010.

———. "Silences and Choice: The Legacies of White Second Wave Feminism in the New Professoriate." *Women's Studies in Communication* 31, no. 2 (July 2008): 143–50. https://doi.org/10.1080/07491409.2008.10162526.

Office of the Chief of Information. "SECNAV Announces New Maternity Leave Policy." *America's Navy*, July 2, 2015. http://www.navy.mil/submit/display.asp?story_id=87987.

Ono, Kent A., and John M. Sloop. "The Critique of Vernacular Discourse." *Communication Monographs* 62, no. 1 (1995): 19–46.

Owen, A. Susan, and Peter Ehrenhaus. "Animating a Critical Rhetoric: On the Feeding Habits of American Empire." *Western Journal of Communication* 57, (Spring 1993): 169–77.
Panzino, Charlsy. "Take Three Years Off: Army Expands Career Intermission Pilot Program." *Army Times*, August 7, 2017. https://www.army times.com/news/your-army/2017/07/09/take-three-years-off-army-expands-career-intermission-pilot-program/.
Pateman, Carole. "The Fraternal Social Contract." In *The Disorder of Women: Democracy, Feminism, and Political Theory*, 33–57. Stanford, CA: Stanford University Press, 1990.
Payne, Deborah, and David A. Nicholls. "Managing Breastfeeding and Work: A Foucauldian Secondary Analysis: Managing Breastfeeding and Work." *Journal of Advanced Nursing* 66, no. 8 (June 16, 2010): 1810–18. https://doi.org/10.1111/j.1365-2648.2009.05156.x.
Peach, Lucinda Joy. "Gender Ideology and the Ethics of Women in Combat." In *It's Our Military Too: Women and the U.S Military*, edited by Judith Stiehm, 156–94. Philadelphia: Temple University Press, 1996.
Pearson, Catherine. "Unplanned Pregnancies among Women in Military High, Rising." *Huffington Post*, January 23, 2013, sec. Women. http://www.huffingtonpost.com/2013/01/23/pregnant-military-unplanned-women_n_2534873.html.
Peters, Rebecca Todd. *Trust Women: A Progressive Christian Argument for Reproductive Justice*. Boston: Beacon Press, 2018.
Pezzullo, Phaedra C. "Performing Critical Interruptions: Stories, Rhetorical Invention, and the Environmental Justice Movement." *Western Journal of Communication* 65, no. 1 (March 2001): 1–25. https://doi.org/10.1080/10570310109374689.
Pierce, Penny F. "The Role of Women in the Military." In *Military Life: Military Culture*, edited by Thomas W. Britt, Amy B. Adler, and Carl Andrew Castro, 97–118. Westport, CT: Greenwood Publishing Group, 2006.
Pittman, Genevra. "Unintended Pregnancies on the Rise in Servicewomen." Reuters. January 24, 2013. http://www.reuters.com/article/2013/01/24/us-pregnancies-servicewoman-idUSBRE90N1B820 130124.
Ponder, Kathryn L., and Melissa Nothnagle. "Damage Control: Unintended Pregnancy in the United States Military." *Journal of Law, Medicine & Ethics* 38, no. 2 (2010): 386–95.

Projansky, Sarah. *Spectacular Girls: Media Fascination and Celebrity Culture*. New York: New York University Press, 2014.
Read, Russel. "Why the US Military is on the Brink of a Recruitment Crisis." WJLA, February 16, 2018. http://wjla.com/news/nation-world/why-the-us-military-is-on-the-brink-of-a-recruitment-crisis.
Reynolds, George M., and Amanda Shendruk. "Demographics of the U.S. Military." Council on Foreign Relations, April 24, 2018. https://www.cfr.org/article/demographics-us-military.
Rich, Adrienne. *Of Woman Born: Motherhood as Experience and Institution*. New York: W. W. Norton & Company, 1995.
Roche-Paull, Robyn, *Breastfeeding in Combat Boots: A Survival Guide to Successful Breastfeeding while Serving in the US Military*. CreateSpace Independent Publish Platform, 2010.
———. "Powerful Photo of Airman Breastfeeding Shows Us What Motherhood in the Military Looks Like." Breastfeeding in Combat Boots, March 8, 2015. http://breastfeedingincombatboots.com/2015/03/powerful-photo-of-airman-breastfeeding-shows-motherhood-military-looks-like/.
Roush, Paul E. "A Tangled Webb the Navy Can't Afford." In *Beyond Zero Tolerance: Discrimination in Military Culture*, edited by Mary Fainsod Katzenstein and Judith Reppy, 81–99. Lanham, MD: Rowman & Littlefield Publishers, 1999.
Rowland, Ashley. "Military Bases Struggle with Breast-Feeding Policies." *Stars and Stripes*, June 18, 2015. https://www.stripes.com/news/pacific/military-bases-struggle-with-breast-feeding-policies-1.352989.
Russell-Kraft, Stephanie. "The Double Standard of Military Pregnancy: What Contraceptive Access Won't Fix." *Rewire News*, August 2, 2016. https://rewire.news/article/2016/08/02/double-standard-military-pregnancy-what-contraceptive-access-wont-fix/.
Sandberg, Sheryl, and Nell Scovall. *Lean In: Women, Work, and the Will to Lead*. New York: Alfred A. Knopf, Inc., 2013.
Schochet, Leila. "The Child Care Crisis Is Keeping Women Out of the Workforce." Center for American Progress, March 28, 2019. https://www.americanprogress.org/issues/early-childhood/reports/2019/03/28/467488/child-care-crisis-keeping-women-workforce/.
Schochet, Leila, and Rasheed Malik. "2 Million Parents Forced to Make Career Sacrifices Due to Problems with Child Care." Center for American Progress, September 13, 2017. https://www.americanprogress.org

/issues/early-childhood/news/2017/09/13/438838/2-million-parents-forced-make-career-sacrifices-due-problems-child-care/.

Schwartz, Felice N. "Management Women and the New Facts of Life." *Women in Management Review* 4, no. 5 (May 1989). https://doi.org/10.1108/EUM0000000001789.

Scott, John Blake. *Risky Rhetoric: AIDS and the Cultural Practices of HIV Testing*. Carbondale: Southern Illinois University Press, 2003.

Sczesny, Sabine, Magda Formanowicz, and Franziska Moser. "Can Gender-Fair Language Reduce Gender Stereotyping and Discrimination?" *Frontiers in Psychology* 7, no. 25 (February 2, 2016). https://doi.org/10.3389/fpsyg.2016.00025.

Selzer, Jack. "Rhetorical Analysis: Understanding How Texts Persuade Readers." In *What Writing Does and How It Does It*, edited by Charles Bazerman and Paul Prior, 279–308. Mahwah, NJ: Lawrence Erlbaum, 2004.

Slaughter, Anne-Marie. *Unfinished Business: Women Men Work Family*. Reprint edition. New York: Random House, 2016.

Smithson, Janet, and Elizabeth H. Stokoe. "Discourses of Work–Life Balance: Negotiating 'Genderblind' Terms in Organizations." *Gender, Work & Organization* 12, no. 2 (2005): 147–68.

Smolinski, Amy Barron. "Military Parental Leave Program-Not Exactly as Promised." MomsRising.org, November 8, 2018. https://www.momsrising.org/blog/military-parental-leave-program-not-exactly-as-promised.

Sonfield, Adam, Kinsey Hasstedt, and Rachel Benson Gold. *Moving Forward: Family Planning in the Era of Health Reform*. Guttmacher Institute, January 27, 2016. https://www.guttmacher.org/report/moving-forward-family-planning-era-health-reform.

Soper, Spencer, and Rebecca Greenfield. "Holdout Jeff Bezos Confronted by Amazon Moms Demanding Day Care." *Bloomberg*, March 4, 2019. https://www.bloomberg.com/news/articles/2019-03-04/holdout-jeff-bezos-confronted-by-amazon-moms-demanding-daycare.

Spelman, Elizabeth V. "Gender & Race: The Ampersand Problem in Feminist Thought." In *Inessential Woman*, 114–209. Boston: Beacon Press, 1988.

Striley, Katie Margavio. "The Stigma of Excellence and the Dialectic of (Perceived) Superiority and Inferiority: Exploring Intellectually Gifted Adolescents' Experiences of Stigma." *Communication Studies* 65, no. 2 (2014): 139–53. http://dx.doi.org/10.1080/10510974.2013.851726.

"Swanson, RADM, Dr. Clifford." https://navy.togetherweserved.com/usn/servlet/tws.webapp.WebApp?cmd=ShadowBoxProfile&type=Person&ID=510505.

Taber, Nancy. "'You Better Not Get Pregnant While You're Here': Tensions between Masculinities and Femininities in Military Communities of Practice." *International Journal of Lifelong Education* 30, no. 3 (June 2011): 331–48. https://doi.org/10.1080/02601370.2011.570871.

Tangney, William. "Recruitment, Retention, and Readiness." *Army Magazine* 49, no. 3 (March 1999): 15.

Tarvis, Carol. *The Mismeasure of Woman: Why Women Are Not the Better Sex, the Inferior Sex, or the Opposite Sex*. New York: Touchstone, 1992.

Thomas, Patricia J., and Marie D. Thomas. "Effects of Sex, Marital Status, and Parental Status on Absenteeism among Navy Enlisted Personnel." *Military Psychology* 6, no. 2 (1994): 95–108.

Tilghman, Andrew, and David Larter. "New 12-Week Maternity Policy for All Services Means Big Cut for Navy, Marines." *Navy Times*, January 28, 2016. http://www.navytimes.com/story/military/2016/01/28/maternity-leave-dod-ash-carter-12-weeks-announcement-force-of-the-future/79465178/.

Time. "The Military Is Pregnant: Coping with Motherhood in the Armed Forces." October 8, 1979.

Titunik, Regina. "Discrimination and Military Culture." *H-Net Reviews*, 2000, 1–3.

Townsley, Nikki C., and Kirsten J. Broadfoot. "Care, Career, and Academe: Heeding the Calls of a New Professoriate." *Women's Studies in Communication* 31, no. 2 (Summer 2008): 133–42. https://doi.org/10.1080/07491409.2008.10162525.

Tracy, Sarah J. *Qualitative Research Methods: Collecting Evidence, Crafting Analysis, Communicating Impact*. Malden, MA: Wiley-Blackwell, 2013.

Truman, Harry S. "Executive Order 10240—Regulations Governing the Separation from the Service of Certain Women Serving in the Regular Army, Navy, Marine Corps, or Air Force." In *The American Presidency Project*, edited by Gerhard Peters and John T. Woolley, April 27, 1951. https://www.presidency.ucsb.edu/documents/executive-order-10240-regulations-governing-the-separation-from-the-service-certain-women.

Truong, Alice. "When Google Increased the Length of Paid Maternity Leave, the Rate New Mothers Quit Dropped by 50%." *Quartz*, January 28, 2016. https://qz.com/604723/when-google-increased-paid-maternity-leave-the-rate-at-which-new-mothers-quit-dropped-50/.

Turner, Paaige K., and Kristen Norwood. "The Elephant in the Room: Negotiating Visible Pregnancy in Job Interviews." *Women & Language* 37, no. 1 (2014): 41–62.

———. "'I Had the Luxury . . .': Organizational Breastfeeding Support as Privatized Privilege." *Human Relations* 67, no. 7 (July 2014): 849–74. https://doi.org/10.1177/0018726713507730.

———. "Unbounded Motherhood: Embodying a Good Working Mother Identity." *Management Communication Quarterly* 27, no. 3 (2013): 396–424.

U.S. Navy. "SECNAV Announces Personnel Initiatives." Navy Live, May 13, 2015. http://navylive.dodlive.mil/2015/05/13/secnav-announces-personnel-initiatives/.

Under Secretary of Defense. "NAVADMIN 151/18: Military Parental Leave Program," June 2018. https://www.public.navy.mil/bupers-npc/reference/messages/Documents/NAVADMINS/NAV2018/NAV18151.txt.

United States Department of Defense. "DoD Instruction 1327.07 Career Intermission Program (CIP) for Service Members," October 18, 2018. https://www.google.com/url?sa=t&rct=j&q=&esrc=s&source=web&cd=5&ved=2ahUKEwjI_8Pj1tXiAhXFg-AKHXg-ALIQFjAEegQIBRAC&url=https%3A%2F%2Fwww.esd.whs.mil%2FPortals%2F54%2FDocuments%2FDD%2Fissuances%2Fdodi%2F132707p.PDF%3Fver%3D2018-10-18-114030-977&usg=AOvVaw189nCrCHHLD-h72CJyueRS.

Vanden Brook, Tom. "Army to Spend $300 Million on Bonuses and Ads to Get 6,000 More Recruits." *USA Today*, February 12, 2017. https://www.usatoday.com/story/news/politics/2017/02/12/army-spend-300-million-bonuses-and-ads-get-6000-more-recruits/97757094/.

Wagner, Brian. "The Military Could Soon Face Increased Recruiting Challenges." *Task and Purpose*, February 18, 2016. https://taskandpurpose.com/the-military-could-soon-face-increased-recruiting-challenges/.

Walters, Joanna. "Yahoo CEO Marissa Mayer's Minimal Maternity Leave Plan Prompts Dismay." *The Guardian*, September 3, 2015, sec. Technology. http://www.theguardian.com/technology/2015/sep/02/yahoo-ceo-marissa-mayer-minimal-maternity-leave-plan-prompts-dismay.

Wattles, Jackie. "Is It Time for Universal Paid Family Leave?" CNN, July 31, 2017. https://money.cnn.com/2017/07/31/news/economy/kirsten-gillibrand-family-act/index.html.

Weiss, Joanna. "Chris Cuomo, Stay in Bed." Politico, April 6, 2020. https://www.politico.com/news/magazine/2020/04/06/chris-cuomo-stay-in-bed-167297.

Whitworth, Sandra. "Militarized Masculinity and Post-Traumatic Stress Disorder." In *Rethinking the Man Question: Sex, Gender and Violence in International Relations*, edited by Jane L. Parpart and Marysia Zalewski, 109–26. London: Zed Books, 2008.

Wilkie, Robert L. "Parental Leave for Military Personnel in Connection with the Birth or Adoption of a Child." March 23, 2018. https://www.med.navy.mil/sites/nmcsd/DocsGME/Policy/MPLP%20Signed%20Policy.pdf.

Wolf, Joan B. *Is Breast Best?: Taking on the Breastfeeding Experts and the New High Stakes of Motherhood*. New York: New York University Press, 2010.

The Women's Armed Services Integration Act of 1948: Public Law No. 80-625, 62 Stat. 368, June 12, 1948. https://www.mcu.usmc.mil/historydivision/Pages/Speeches/PublicLaw625.aspx.

World Health Organization. "WHO Recommendation on Midwife-Led Continuity of Care during Pregnancy," November 1, 2016. https://extranet.who.int/rhl/topics/improving-health-system-performance/implementation-strategies/who-recommendation-midwife-led-continuity-care-during-pregnancy.

Yarrow, Allison. "Shaheen Amendment Expands Female Service Members' Access to Abortion." *The Daily Beast*, January 3, 2013. http://www.thedailybeast.com/articles/2013/01/03/shaheen-amendment-expands-female-service-members-access-to-abortion.html.

Young, Iris Marion. *On Female Body Experience "Throwing Like a Girl" and Other Essays*. New York: Oxford University Press, 2005.

Zaeske, Susan. *Signatures of Citizenship: Petitioning, Antislavery, and Women's Political Identity*. Chapel Hill: University of North Carolina Press, 2003.

Index

ableism, 79
abortion, 43
absenteeism, 10, 119
abstinence-only deployments policy, 27
academic careers, 111-12, 156
accommodations and guidelines: for breastfeeding, 119-20; ignoring, 92-94, 97, 113-15, 117-18; importance of taking, 160; using to transition to work, 123; women advising women to use, 95-96
Acker, Joan, 101
Additional Maternity Leave (AML), Navy, 109
age for pregnancy, 55-56, 68, 111
Air Force: breastmilk pumping in, 128-29; Career Intermission Program (CIP) in, 35, 37, 67; diversity and inclusion initiatives of, 8; image of servicewomen breastfeeding, 1-2, 2*fig*; images of breastfeeding in uniform, 149, 149*fig*; interviews with servicewomen, 35; maternity jumper, *82*; military maternity uniforms in, 81

Alexa, Air Force officer: maternity uniforms, 81, 82-83; military healthcare, 85; as minority in military, 90; resisting macho maternity, 95-96; unplanned pregnancy, 58
Amazon (company), 131
Ames, Genevieve M., 10, 59
appendicitis, pregnancy compared to, 73
Apple (company), 131
Ariel, Navy sailor, 50, 91, 93, 94
Army: Army Nurse Corps Auxiliary, 28; Career Intermission Program (CIP) in, 35; deployment schedules in, 50; uniform changes in, 153; Women's Army Auxiliary Corps (WAAC), 25
Army Combat Uniform-Alternate, 153
Ashcraft, Karen Lee, 101
assertiveness, 3
assumptions: about pregnancy, 45, 47; about pregnancy and work, 78, 97; challenging, 157; linked to women, 103, 141, 151; man as normal, 15-16, 33, 44-45, 97, 101; unpinning culture, 20-21

239

athletes, professional, 112
attrition rates of women, 67
auxiliary roles of women in military, 27–28
aviators, career paths of, 52, 67

banking and accounting professions, 89
barriers to service, 25, 32
bathrooms, pumping breastmilk in, 128–29
Beall, Jade, 148, 149
bed rest, 91
Benya, Frazier F., 16–17, 20, 21
Bezos, Jeff, 131
Biggs, R. Lee, 10, 16
binary, male-female, 11, 12
biological sex differences, 74, 76, 80, 89
birth control. *See* contraception
birthing, 87, 90–93
Blair-Loy, Mary, 101, 137–38
bodies: biological realities of, 56; changes during pregnancy, 92; changes from pregnancy, 45, 73–74; disciplining female, 14, 44–45, 48, 57, 59; female as different, 10, 11, 33; hysterization of female, 74; inferiority of female, 74, 76; lactating, 126; maternal integration into military, 31–38; military focus on availability of, 159; moral standards applied to female, 26; pathologizing female, 16; pregnant violating uniformity, 94; White male as normal, 15–16, 70, 101
body fat test, 46–47, 109
bounded motherhood, 104
breastfeeding: duration recommendations for, 121; frequency of, 99–100; health benefits of, 119, 120, 127; images of, 1–2, 2*fig*, 3–4, *147*, 148, 149*fig*; policies for, 37–38; intensive mothering ideologies in, 118–19; marginalization of in workplace, 127; mastitis, 71; public conversations about, 146; supportive culture at Pentagon, 129–30
"breast is best" ideas, 118
breastmilk production, 100, 125
breastmilk pumping: accommodations for in workplace, 119; balancing with job, 122, 124, 126; challenges of, 122;
embarrassment about, 127; frequency of, 99–100; locations for, 128; policies regulating in 1990s, 37–38; pressure to avoid at work, 124–25; self-advocacy in, 130; space for in Navy, 121; successful stories of at work, 123, 129–30; time consumption of at work, 125; traveling while, 76–77
Broadfoot, Kirsten J., 156
broken leg, pregnancy compared to, 73–74
Brooks, Rosa, 156–57
Brown, Melissa T., 38
Buchanan, Lindal, 101-2, 104
Bureau of Labor Statistics, 105
Burke, Carol, 22
Buzzanell, Patrice M., 10, 48, 79, 104, 115

Candee, Navy officer: childcare challenges, 131; guilt about maternity leave, 64–65; medicalizing pregnancy, 73; mentoring, 144; military medical care, 86; serving in Reserves, 67; work-life balance, 162–63
career flexibility, increasing, 106–7, 108, 115–16, 119–20
Career Intermission Program (CIP), 35–37, 67–68, 123
career progression: for aviators, 52; Career Intermission Program (CIP), 35; challenges in aviation and pregnancy, 91; choices around, 136–37; concerns about disrupting, 40, 49–52, 60; decisions made with women's input, 76–77; military masculinity mindset, 12; promotion schedules, 35–36, 66, 113; time off as a threat to, 111–12; women in top ranks, 157, 162
Carter, Ash (Secretary of Defense), 110, 112, 152
Cesarean sections (C-sections), 87, 116
chain of command, 41, 75, 78
challenging discourses, 21, 70, 96–98, 155
Cheney, George, 6–7
childcare: expanded services, 145; quality in military, 109, 123; recommendations for improving, 161; responsibility of women, 118; struggles, 130–33
Child Development Center (CDC), 131, 132, 145

INDEX 241

choices: based on health of children, 138; to be in military, 69–70; constrained, 61–62, 135–36; emphasis on personal, 12–13; hyperplanning pregnancies, 41, 48; impression of, 139; lack of around pregnancy, 62; rhetoric of, 57, 66, 70, 83, 135–36; second wave feminism emphasis on, 103

Cindy, Navy officer: avoiding difference, 71; breastfeeding, 120; breastmilk pumping, 128; job selection, 66; maternity uniforms, 81; personal choices, 136–37; pregnancy planning, 58; pregnancy stigma, 45; supermom identity, 140; working until birth, 91

Clarissa, Air Force servicewoman, 69, 75–76, 78, 128

Claudia, Navy officer: breastfeeding and pumping at work, 123; breastmilk drying up, 125; career path, 52; job pressures and breastfeeding, 126; maternity leave length, 114; medicalization of pregnancy, 73; pregnancy planning, 50–51, 54, 58; training while breastfeeding, 117

Clementine, Air Force officer: breastfeeding, 120; Career Intermission Program (CIP), 35, 67–68, 123; career progression, 53; childcare challenges, 132, 133; places to pump at work, 128–29; pregnancy as problem, 37; unplanned pregnancy, 58–59

co-constructors of discourse, women as, 70, 72, 88, 113

colleagues, pressure from, 41, 54, 78, 81, 130

Collett, Jessica L., 103

combat, women in, 6, 23, 27

combat readiness: pregnancy not affecting, 68; pregnancy perceived as affecting, 9–10, 18, 26, 30, 32, 45

commanding officers (CO), 61, 76–77, 97, 161

commitment: to child rearing, 116; to military, 64–65, 141; mutual, 108

communication studies, 6

community vs. individualism, 12–13, 115–16

condoms. See contraception

contraception, 26, 42–43, 51, 57–59, 69

contradictory cultures, 10–15, 44, 96, 103, 112, 113

control: fertility, 18, 41–42, 64, 159; lack of in health care decisions, 84–88; of personal lives, 30; underpinning force in military, 59, 63, 64, 66, 68

convalescent leave, 80, 150, 151

corporate paternalism, 50, 57

COVID-19, 112

Crawford, Stephanie, 31–32

critical feminist orientation, 5, 6, 19, 21

cultural change: efficacy of language change in, 151; men's role in, 157; movement toward, 15–21, 158–64; women's role in, 12

cultural tensions, 10–15, 30. See also tensions

Cunico, Jonea (Staff Sergeant), 146–47, 147fig

Cuomo, Chris (CNN journalist), 112

Defense Advisory Committee to Women in the Services (DACOWITS), 153

Defense Officer Personnel Management Act (DOPMA), 111–12

delaying child birth, 64, 111

D'Enbeau, Suzy, 48

Department of Defense, 35, 109, 119, 150, 151

dependents, military, health care of, 86

deployment: abstinence-only policy, 27; accusations of avoiding, 18, 26, 40–41, 44–47; deferred after childbirth, 113; policies, 62–63; pregnant women excluded from, 158–59; waiving deferred, 117, 145

difference, avoidance of, 93, 101, 104, 151, 153, 155

disability, pregnancy as, 76, 78, 79–80, 150

disability leave, short-term, 79, 105–6

discipline, circuits of: avoiding postpartum benefits, 113, 116; conforming to ideal servicemember expectations, 88, 100; hyperplanning pregnancy, 68–69; ways to break, 145, 154–55

discipline of bodies, 14, 15, 44–45, 48

discourses: around motherhood, 9; around parenthood, 155; definitions,

discourses (*continued*)
  5, 6; maternity leave, 118; neoliberal, 13–17; post-feminist, 139; pregnancy planning, 43–44
discrimination against women in military: discrimination responses of military, 7–8, 16; experienced as stigma, 44–47; history of, 28–29; morally superior argument for, 25–27; persistence of, 18–20; pregnancy and, 14, 20, 24, 44–47; unconstitutional, 24; women held responsible for, 13
diversity and inclusion initiatives, 8, 152–53
doctors, military, 42, 59, 71–72, 85–86
Douglas, Susan, 102, 115, 140
draft end, 32
dual career families, 130–31, 137
Duke, Michael R., 10, 59

Echegoyen-McCabe, Terran, 2, 2*fig*, 146
egg-freezing, 68, 110, 111
Elizabeth, Navy public affairs officer: childcare waitlists, 132; cultural change in military, 146, 155, 157–58; dual-career families, 137; experience at the Pentagon, 129–30; family planning, 64; gender-neutral pay scales, 8; maternity leave, 113; maternity uniforms, 81, 83; mentoring, 143; physical readiness tests (PRT), 134; postpartum depression, 140–41; pride of suffering trope, 117; prioritizing family, 65, 66; shiftwork and childcare, 133; turning down accommodations, 92–93; uniforms, 34; unplanned pregnancy, 59, 61–62
Ellingson, Laura L., 10, 79
Elsa, Navy officer: career path, 52; pregnancy as disability, 78–79; breastmilk pumping, 122, 128; health of children in choices, 138–39; mentoring, 143; taking maternity leave, 114–15; pregnancy planning, 50, 53; prioritizing family, 64, 65
Emily, Navy servicewoman, 83, 85, 87–88, 116
Enloe, Cynthia, 11, 16, 38
executive officers (XO), 61, 64

Executive Order 10240, 29, 31
Eyer, Diane, 103

Facebook, 3, 154
familiarization trips, 76–77
family leave, paid, 105–6
Family Medical Leave Act (FMLA), 105–6
family planning. *See* fertility planning
fathers as secondary caregivers, 152
female embodiment, 11, 12. *See also* bodies
femininity, 11, 34
feminism, 38, 103, 118–19, 139
fertility control, 18, 41–42, 64, 159
fertility planning, 9, 45, 49–53, 64
Fifth Amendment to the Constitution of the United States, 24
Fixmer-Oraiz, Natalie, 13–14, 21, 22, 102
Fleet Week, 99, 100, 114
flexibility of jobs, 66, 75–76, 158
Flores, Anna, 23
Flores v. Secretary of Defense, 23–24
footwear, 93–94
Force of the Future initiative, 110
Foucault, Michel, 13–14, 74, 88
Fourteenth Amendment of the Constitution of the United States, 32
fraternity, 11
freezing breastmilk, 121
Frida, Navy officer: accommodations for pregnancy, 94; deployment after pregnancy, 62–63; macho maternity leave, 113–14; breastmilk pumping, 124, 125; deployment after birth, 117; experience at the Pentagon, 130; mentoring, 143–44; resistance to intensive mothering, 142–43, 155; pregnancy planning, 58; prioritizing family, 64; resisting macho maternity, 95

genderblind military, 34, 151
gender equality, 8, 11–12, 33, 68, 89
gender-neutrality: Career Intermission Program (CIP), 37; gender-neutral terms, 49, 150–51, 152; goal of uniforms, 83–84; goal of uniforms, 10, 33; of ideal workers, 101
gender roles and scripts, traditional, 14, 89, 102

Getoya, Navy officer: childcare challenges, 132; judgment from women about maternity leave, 117; lack of support from women, 126; maternity uniforms, 81; promotion and pregnancy, 51–52; rhetoric of choice, 66–67; stigma around pregnancy, 46; working until birth, 91
good mother identities, 118, 122–24, 126, 139–40
good worker identities, 113–15, 118, 122–24, 126, 139–40, 164
good working mothers, 103, 104, 108, 113, 137, 139–40
Google, 109, 131
grandparents for childcare, 132–33
Grumet, Jamie Lynne, 1
Guenter-Schlesinger, Sue, 16
guidelines and accommodations: ignoring, 92–94, 113, 117, 118; importance of taking, 160; women advising women to use, 95–96
Guide 8 (Navy pregnancy guide), 80
guilt, 54, 64, 143, 159–60
Gutmann, Stephanie, 73
gynecologists, 86

Haraway, Donna, 6
Hayden, Sara, 13, 141
Hays, Sharon, 31, 102, 103, 137
healing from birthing, 116, 135
health care, reproductive, 71–72
health care providers, military: lack of continuity in, 85–86, 98; military dependents, care for, 86; recommendations to improve, 160; regulation of, 75; reproductive, 71–72; restrictions on, 87
hierarchy, 20, 21, 87
Holm, Jeanne, 29, 30
Holt, Kelsey, 41
homeland maternity, 13–15, 102
hypermasculinity, culture of, 10–13, 21, 33, 144, 158, 163–64. *See also* masculinity
hyperplanning pregnancies: attitudes toward birth control, 42–43; expectations of Navy for, 50–53; failures of, 57–63; frustration about, 55–57; lack of privacy in, 63–64; military responses to resistance to, 67–68; reporting pregnancies, 40–41; resisting, 63–67, 154; as response to stigma, 47–49; statistics on planned *vs.* unplanned pregnancies, 41–42; women's responsibility in, 53–55
hysterization of female bodies, 74. *See also* bodies

ideal service members, 94, 100–101
identities: construction of, 105, 114; dual, 108; good mother, 118, 122–24, 126, 139–40; good worker, 113–15, 118, 122–24, 126, 139–40, 164; good working mother, 103–4, 108, 113, 137, 139–40; importance of, 104
identities, intersectional, 89, 96, 100
images, controversial, 1–2, 2*fig*, 146–47
inclusion of family diversity in policies, 152–53
individual responsibility, 12–13, 103, 118, 139, 140. *See also* responsibilization
informing *vs.* asking permission about pregnancy, 64, 69, 75–76, 92
Instructions, the: breastfeeding, 119; breastmilk pumping, 128; convalescent leave, 80; ignoring, 94; introduction, 48–49; in-vitro fertilization, 63, 64; language in, 150
insurance, military, 63, 69, 84, 156
intensive mothering ideology: breastfeeding as part of, 118, 126; good working mother identity, 137, 139; as institutionalized motherhood, 102, 103; introduction, 31; resistance to, 142; ubiquity required for, 157
intersections between cultures, 10–15
interuterine device (IUD), 58
interviews, 5–6, 7, 44
invasiveness of hyperplanning pregnancies, 63–64
in vitro fertilization (IVF), 55–56, 63–64
involuntary separations, 8–9, 29–32, 44
Ivette, Navy servicewoman, 85
Ivie, Robert L., 21, 22

Jada, Navy sailor, 46, 56, 83
Joanna, Army servicewoman, 91, 123

Johnson, Paula A., 16–17, 20, 21
judgment. *See* stigma
Jules, junior enlisted sailor, 46, 72, 85, 87
junior officers, 56–57

Katzenstein, Mary Fainsod, 16
Kimmel, Michael S., 11
knowledge, social construction of, 6
Koerber, Amy, 118–19, 127, 144
Kornfield, Sarah, 79
Kosloski, Sandy, *82*
Kristen, Navy officer, 91, 115, 134, 136, 143

labor of women undervalued, 95, 127
Lair, Daniel J., 6–7
language, 69, 79–80, 108, 152
Lean In movement, 156
Luna, Christina, 2, 2*fig*, 146
Lundquist, Jennifer Hickes, 9
Lynn, Air Force officer, 77; breastmilk, 125, 129; childcare challenges, 132; footwear, 93; lack of support from women, 126; maternity leave perceptions, 116; pregnancy as disability, 79; punishment for pregnancy, 77–78; resistance, 136; separation of work and mother spheres, 127; on Training Duty (TDY) with infant, 117; women as minority, 129; working until birth, 91

Mabus, Ray (Secretary of Navy), 33, 106–7, 108, 115, 159
macho maternity: defined, 89; ignoring accommodations, 92–94; introduction, 71, 88–89; maternity leave, 112–18; not taking all maternity leave, 114–15; resisting, 95–96, 143, 153–58; as response to ideal worker assumptions, 101; working until birth, 90–92
Mack, Ashley N., 15, 102
Mae, Navy officer: breastfeeding, 120; experience at the Pentagon, 130; gratitude for maternity policies, 123; hyperplanning pregnancies, 40; leaving military, 67; maternity leave, 108–9; military maternity policies, 8, 54–55; rank and privacy, 75; sea-to-shore rotations, 51; stigma, 45; work-life balance difficulties, 157

Magellan, Navy servicewoman: intersectional identities, 89; sea-to-shore rotations, 53–54; women in combat, 23; working twice as hard as men, 90–91; reporting her pregnancy, 92
male-dominated organizations, 3, 17, 131, 138
male-female binary, 11, 12
man as normal assumptions, 15–16, 33, 44–45, 97, 101
Marine Corps, 28, 31–32, 107, 108, 109, 150–51
marriage, 137, 143–44
Martin, Joanne, 50, 142
Mary, Navy servicewoman, 75
masculinity: definitions, 11, 20; masculinizing women, 34; as norm, 33, 44–45; military, 12; and work, 101
Master Sergeant Mom, 84
mastitis, 71
maternal age, advanced, 55–56, 111
maternal behavior, appropriate, 1, 3, 9, 44, 49
maternal bodies. *See* bodies
"maternal wall," 78
maternity as problem culture, 4, 10, 15–16, 55–56. *See also* pregnancy as problem culture
Maternity Convalescent leave, 152
maternity leave: as disability leave, 79; duration, 99, 106–7, 110; eighteen week leave in Navy, 106–8, 110, 111; generous in military, 100; health benefits of paid, 107–8; importance of taking, 160; not taking all of, 116, 118; perceptions as vacation, 116; policies, 105–12; promotions while on, 113–14; rate of paid in U.S., 105; term use changes, 150–51. *See also* convalescent leave; family leave, paid; maternity policies in the military
maternity policies in the military: in Air Force, 8; breastfeeding and pumping, 119–20; evolution in, 150–52, 160–61; examples of, 4; exemplary, 16, 39, 43; as generous, 100; introduction of after September 11, 2001, 6, 7; invasive, 69; negotiating, 88; newer policies, 152–53; paid leave, 106–7; term use

changes, 150–51. *See also* breastfeeding; breastmilk pumping; maternity leave
maternity uniforms. *See* uniforms, military
Maucione, Scott, 36
Mayer, Marissa, 3, 154
McCarver, Virginia, 139
medical files, 75
medicalization of pregnancy, 72–76, 79
Meisenbach, Rebecca, 88, 118
men: erasure of role of in pregnancies, 69; as ideal workers, 27, 70, 155; lack of stigma in family planning, 68; man as normal assumptions, 15–16, 33, 44–45, 97, 101; role of in reproductive planning, 9; White, 101; work-life balance, 162
mentoring, 142–45, 161–63
Meyer, Marissa, 113
Michaels, Meredith, 102, 115, 140
Michelle, retired Navy officer: freezing eggs, 68; gender equality in military, 8; mastitis, 71–72; military schedules and pregnancy, 60; paternalistic attitudes, 76–77; pregnancy continuum experience, 7, 22; pumping breastmilk, 121–22, 128–29; rank and motherhood, 137; responsibility and guilt, 54
micropractices, 48, 68, 88, 154
midwives, 84–85, 86, 97–98
military, leaving, 67, 157, 162
military, reasons for joining, 95
Military Abortion Amendment, 43
military culture: around maternity, 19; discriminatory, 23; hypermasculinity, 11–12, 21, 33, 144, 158, 163–64; of individualization, 12–13; promoting social change in, 7–10
military health care system. *See* health care providers, military
Military Medicine, 9
military policies, influence on public policies, 18, 38, 109, 110, 163
military policy discourse, 93–94
military schedules and structures: conforming to, 49–54, 126; changes in, 60–63; high regulation of, 75
military termination criteria for women, 29–30

military treatment facilities (MTF), 87
milk loss, 125
Miranda, Navy officer: birth control, 26, 42–43; privacy, 75; pumping breastmilk, 99–100; shipping breastmilk, 121–22; taking maternity leave, 114
miscarriages, 40, 59
Mom2Mom support group, 2
moral standards, 23–27, 42, 43
mother as "god term," 102
motherhood: bounded or unbounded, 104; cultural understandings of, 101–2; innateness to women, 29–31; language around, 108; mothers, 103; responsibility of, 45; as termination criteria, 29–30

Natalie, enlisted Navy sailor: career aspirations, 40; physical readiness tests (PRT), 135; pregnancy reporting, 69; reproductive health care, 75, 85; role of men in sex, 9
National Compensation Survey, 105
National Public Radio, *Morning Edition*, 109
national security, 13–14
Navy: breastfeeding in, 119, 120–21; Career Intermission Program (CIP), 35–37; contraception in, 26, 43; health care in, 71–72; maternity leave expansion, 106–7, 150; maternity uniform, 81, *82*; number of women in, 109; pregnancy in, 23–24, 47–49; rates of pregnancy in, 72; Reserves, 28; sea and shore rotations in, 49–53; servicewomen as focus of research, 6; women's uniforms, 33–34; working twice as hard in, 90
Navy Office of Women's Policy, 49
neoliberalism: discourses of, 88; emphasis on control, 48; introduction, 12–13; in macho maternity, 118; in military culture, 15; rhetoric of choice and, 16, 139; underpinning bringing children to work, 115
new momism, 102
Nicholls, David A., 124, 127
"Normalize Breastfeeding" project, 148–49

norms of bodies, 15–16, 70. *See also* bodies
Norwood, Kristen, 104, 126
nurses in military, 28

objectivity, 74–75
O'Brien Hallstein, D. Lynn, 13, 101–2, 103, 140, 141
obstetricians, 62, 85, 98
operations officers, 60–61
OPNAV 6001.C, 48–49, 62, 119, 120–21, 124, 133
OPNAV 6001.D, 150, 151
organizational climate *vs.* culture, 20, 126
organizations, male-dominated, 3, 17, 96, 131, 137–38, 151

Paige, Navy officer: breastmilk pumping, 125, 126; child health and choices, 138; dual-career families, 137; experiences at the Pentagon, 130; mentoring, 143–44; paternalistic attitudes, 76–77; pregnancy planning, 51, 58; promotion schedules, 66, 113, 137; reproductive health care, 85; stigma of breastmilk pumping, 127–28
parental and paternity leave, 152
parenthood discourses, 155
Pateman, Carole, 11
paternalistic and patronizing attitudes, 76–80
pathologizing pregnancy, 72–73, 76–77, 161
patriarchy, 3, 21, 79, 139
Payne, Deborah, 124, 127
pay scale, gender- and race-neutral, 8
Pentagon, 129–30, 132
Pezzullo, Phaedra C., 7
photos of breastfeeding, 1–2, 2*fig*, 146–47, 148
physical readiness to return to work, 133–35
physical training (PT) and tests, 46–47, 94, 109
pilots, 52, 56, 67
Plate, Admiral, 24
policy/culture disconnect: around pregnancy planning, 43, 54; breastmilk pumping, 126–27; discriminatory barriers contributing to, 25; introduction, 4; in military regarding pregnancy, 18–20; sexual harassment example, 16–17; steps to resolve, 163–64; strength of cultural influences, 70
post-feminist discourse, 13, 16, 139
postpartum period: behaviors, 113; challenges, 141; deferment waiver, 62; depression symptoms (PDS), 140–41; experiences, 112; policies, 37–38; recovery time, 116. *See also* breastfeeding; breastmilk pumping; maternity leave
post-traumatic stress disorder (PTSD), 87–88
powerlessness in health care decisions, 84–88. *See also* health care providers, military
pregnancies: age and planning, 55–56; body changes from, 45, 116; emotionality of, 73; health care during, 84–88; importance of planning, 51; job type importance in planning, 52; long-term effects of, 73–74; overlooking unplanned, 111; planned *vs.* unplanned, 18; rates of, 41–42, 46, 47, 83; regulation of in military, 75; reporting, 24–25, 40–41, 160–61; seen as avoidance of military obligations, 24, 40, 41, 44; seen as deviation from norm, 10, 16; seen as irresponsible, 62; stigma, 44–47; symptoms, 92; variables of, 44, 48, 55
pregnancy as problem culture: despite policies, 16; historical context of, 32–33; introduction, 8–10; medicalization of pregnancy, 72–74; pregnancy to avoid work, 44–45; reinforcing of, 37, 68–69, 97, 154
prenatal care in military, 97–98
pressures: to be capable, 89; from colleagues, 54; as a minority, 90, 100, 114–15; resisting cultural, 142–44
Primary Caregiver Leave (PCL), 152
priorities, 64–66, 162–63
privacy, lack of, 63–64, 75–76
professional advancement. *See* career progression; promotion timelines
professionalism, impressions of, 54, 81, 114–15

promotion timelines, 35–36, 66, 113, 136–37. *See also* career progression
public affairs officers, 42, 52, 59, 92, 99
public policies, influenced by military policies, 18, 38, 109, 110, 163
public/private sphere conflation, 25, 27, 31, 75–76, 103–4, 142
public relations officers, 66
punishment for pregnancy, 62, 83–84, 97

qualitative methods, 6. *See also* research methods

racial integration, 8
rank: breastfeeding, 123; maternity leave length, 114; motherhood, 137; pregnancy pressure, 92; pregnancy privacy, 75; pregnancy stigma, 45–46
rape in military, 42
readiness, combat: constant maintenance of, 59; planned pregnancies to improve, 49, 57, 70; pregnancy as disability, 80; pregnancy impact on, 9–10, 68; research on pregnancy impact on, 18; retention stabilizing, 107; stigma, 45
Reagan administration, 9
recommendations for change, 96–98, 144–45, 158, 160–64
recruitment of women: after September 11, 2001, 6; beginning in 1970s, 32; crisis in, 13–14; as a goal of military, 159; policies to improve, 8, 106–7, 109, 110, 131
reinforcing discriminating discourses: how to avoid, 160; rhetoric of choice, 139; synthesis, 154–55; through macho maternity, 88–89, 96, 100, 116, 118
relationships in military, 43
replacability, 64–65
Reppy, Judith, 16
reproductive planning. *See* fertility planning
reproductive rights in United States, 70
research methods, 4–7
research project, origins, 4
Reserves, 28, 67, 144, 146, 148, 162
resistance: to intensive mothering, 63–67; of macho maternity, 95–96, 136, 153–58; mentoring as, 142–44

responsibilization: culture of, 17, 24; in hyperplanning pregnancies, 53–55; influence on choices, 115; introduction, 12–13; in "leaning in," 156; women reinforcing, 47–48, 68–69, 139, 144, 154
retention of women: Career Intermission Program (CIP) for, 35; as a goal of military, 159; in higher ranks, 158; maternity leave length, 109–10; policies for, 9–10, 131; rank and motherhood, 162; struggles in, 19–20
retirement, 134, 138, 162–63
rhetoric: analysis, 4, 5, 7; of choice, 135, 136; problem view, 21; of reproduction, 15; of supermom identities, 141
Rich, Adrienne, 102
Roche-Paull, Robyn, *Breastfeeding in Combat Boots*, 37–38, 148
role-modeling to other servicewomen, 95–96
Roxanne, Navy officer: childcare challenges, 133; flying while pregnant, 91; in-vitro fertilization, 55–56, 63–64; military health care regulation, 85, 86; pressure to work harder, 89–90; resistance to intensive mothering, 142
Ruby, Tara, 148, 149, 149*fig*

Sadie, Navy officer, 50, 57, 67, 81, 137, 162
Samantha, junior enlisted sailor, 91
Sandberg, Sheryl, 154
Sandberg, Sheryl, *Lean In*, 3, 156
schedules, deployment, 49–54. *See also* military schedules and structures
schemas, 101
science, 73, 74, 109, 127
sea duty, 49–53, 55–56, 60
SEAL teams, 60, 71
sea-to-shore rotations, 49–53, 60–61
Secondary Caregiver Leave (SCL), 152
self-disciplining to meet expectations, 88
selfishness, 65
separation of men and women, 25
separations, involuntary, 8–9, 29–32, 44
September 11, 2001, 6, 13–14
Servello, Chris, (Navy Commander), 109
servicewomen's input into decisions, 162
sex, women's responsibility for, 26–27

sexism, 45
sexual harassment, 16, 21
sheros (she+heros), 148
shiftwork, 145
shipping breastmilk, 121–22
shore duty, 49–53, 64
short-term disability plans, 105–6
Simmons, Vanessa, 149
situated knowledges, 6
Slaughter, Anne-Marie, 117, 154
Smith, Herbert L., 9
Smithson, Janet, 89, 101, 151
smoking breaks, 127–28
snowball sampling, 6. *See also* research methods
social media, 2
stakeholder voices, 4, 21
stay-at-home mothers, 103
stigma: about contraception, 42; about maternity leave, 117; around pumping breastmilk, 127–28; hyperplanning pregnancy to avoid, 54, 56–57, 61; against pregnancy, 44–47; techniques to avoid, 136; of using accommodations policies, 97; women reinforcing, 88
Stokoe, Elizabeth H., 89, 101, 151
stress from fitting into military schedules, 59, 132, 133
striving for success, 65–66
supermom identities, 139–43
surface warfare officers (SWO), 99, 126
Swanson, Clifford A. (Rear Admiral), 30
Sydney, Navy servicewoman, 78
symbols, 5
systems: systemic change, 158–64; systemic problem view, 20, 139, 145, 156, 157–58; systemic responsibility, 103, 139, 141

Tanya, Navy servicewoman, 60–61, 66, 78–79, 84–85, 141
technology and science careers, 109
telecommuting, 3
tensions: community *vs.* individual, 115–16; cultural, 10–15; gender equality *vs.* biological sex differences, 89, 100; good mother *vs.* good worker, 101–5
tenure, 111–12

termination criteria for women in military, 29–30. *See also* involuntary separations
Thomas, Marie D., 10
Thomas, Patricia J., 10
"three Rs," 9–10. *See also* readiness, combat; retention of women
Time magazine, 1, 9
time off, fear of taking, 111–12
tokenism, 157–58
Townsley, Nikki C., 156
Training Duty (TDY), 117, 136
transition back to work, 99, 108–9, 115, 123, 131–32
trauma, from birthing, 87
Truman, Harry S., 29, 31
Turner, Paaige K., 104, 126

ubiquity, required for intensive mothering, 157
unbounded motherhood, 104
uniformity, importance of, 93–94, 97
uniforms, military: breastfeeding in, 2, 2*fig*, 3–4, 146, 148, 149*fig*; changes in the Army, 153; contradictions in purpose, 83–84; fitting into after pregnancy, 135; gender neutral, 10, 33–35; maternity, 81–83, 82*fig*, 97; pants style, 81–82; as punishment, 80–84; unisex alternate, 153; women's Navy, 34
unpaid labor, 47, 95
U.S. lacking paid family leave, 105

victim-blaming, 54
volunteerism in military, 69–70

waitlists for childcare, 132–33, 145
Waldfogel, Jane, 109
Weiss, Joanna, 112
Widnall, Sheila E., 16–17, 20, 21
Wolf, Joan B., 118
women: in combat, 6, 23, 27; historical roles in military, 27–29, 34; as innately mothers, 29–31; labor of undervalued, 47, 95; as minorities in military, 90, 158; as negative in military, 116; as professionally inferior, 27–29, 76; recruitment of, 6, 8, 13–14,

Founded in 1893,
UNIVERSITY OF CALIFORNIA PRESS
publishes bold, progressive books and journals
on topics in the arts, humanities, social sciences,
and natural sciences—with a focus on social
justice issues—that inspire thought and action
among readers worldwide.

The UC PRESS FOUNDATION
raises funds to uphold the press's vital role
as an independent, nonprofit publisher, and
receives philanthropic support from a wide
range of individuals and institutions—and from
committed readers like you. To learn more, visit
ucpress.edu/supportus.

INDEX 249

work-life balance: breastmilk pumping as example, 130; Career Intermission Program (CIP) to support, 35–37; difficulty of, 66–67, 103–4, 109; effects on men, 162; harder after birthing, 135; Lean In movement and, 156; personal differences in, 78; responsibilization in, 118; rhetoric surrounding, 70; supermoms, 140
World Breastfeeding Week, 2
World Health Organization, 121
World War II, 31

Yahoo, 3, 113, 154
Young, 74

32, 34; responsibility of for sex, 26–27; retention of, 9–10, 19–20, 35; role of in reproductive planning, 9; separation of from men, 25
Women Accepted for Voluntary Emergency Service (WAVES), 25–26
Women's Armed Services Act (WASIA), 28, 29
Women's Army Auxiliary Corps (WAAC), 25–26
work: efforts of men and women, 89; ethic, 78, 112; maternity culture in workplaces, 20; pressure to work harder, 89–92; women in workplaces, 31; working mothers, 3

www.ingramcontent.com/pod-product-compliance
Lightning Source LLC
Chambersburg PA
CBHW030535230426

4366SCB00010B/904